EVEN DOCTORS CRY

Love, Death, Scandal and a Terribly Flawed Medical System

A Beverly Hills
Plastic Surgeon's Story

Alvin Reiter, MD

Langdon Street Press
212 3rd Avenue North, Suite 290
Minneapolis, MN 55401
612.455.2293
www.langdonstreetpress.com

ISBN - 978-1-936183-05-0
ISBN - 1-936183-05-6
LCCN - 2009940145

Typeset in Garamond by Melanie Shellito

Printed in the United States of America

Dedication

To my loving wife Nancy, who encouraged and helped me to write this book, but even more, showed grace under fire — my fire and moods. Thank you for staying the course. I truly love you.

And to all those medical professionals who through communication with their patients, develop understanding, diminish fear and keep hope alive. And to all those faced with the dilemma of life-threatening disease, to successfully navigate the physical, mental, emotional and spiritual aspects of cancer.

Acknowledgements

Without the following people, there would have been no book:

My medical fraternity, Phi Delta Epsilon, whose members upon first hearing my story, told me "it sounds like a book." And now it is.

Dr. Elizabeth Trawick who patiently listend to my story again and again and painstakingly pointed me in the direction of seeing the glass half full.

My brother Ira and my sister-in-law Suzyn, for always being there for me.

Dr. Dave Hoffman, our outstanding oncologist, for helping Karen traverse the final steps of life's journey.

Beanie, Cecil, Pearlie, Blackie, Stanley and RIP Wojge, Dexter, Tinker and Doodle in cat heaven, whose soft purrs are truly the sweetest sounds this side of heaven.

Esther Padilla, *muchas gracias por todo, que Dias los bendiga.*

And the many others whose compassion and kindness during my difficult days I will never forget.

Contents

Chapter One

BEVERLY HILLS DOC

L iving in Beverly Hills can lull you into a false sense of security. Los Angeles may be one of the crime capitals of the world, with gang wars, drive-by shootings, race riots and road rage. However, for most of the upper middle class who inhabit the fertile crescent of fame, wealth and power that winds its palm-shaded way west from Beverly Hills to Malibu, crime—violent crime, as opposed to being bankrupted by one's business manager, and with the exception of the O.J. Simpson case—is something that happens so far to the east that it might as well occur on another planet, or on television. Thus, it was quite shocking to me on a quiet night in 1997 to be woken up at my own Bel Air home to do emergency surgery on a young man and his girlfriend whose throats had been slashed by assailants. The crime had taken place at their residence "north of Montana," which isn't in the Rockies but, rather, in the most desirable and most stratospherically priced precinct of nearby Santa Monica.

As a surgeon, I wasn't shocked by much—I had cut my teeth on the aftermath of violent crime—but when it hits so close to home, your it-can't-happen-to-me complacency gets challenged. But this was a red alert situation, with no time for reflection on sociology or the efficiency of the neighborhood patrol. My wife, Karen, was inured after fifteen years of such midnight crises. She was a sound sleeper, and I didn't want to disturb her, but then I thought I might be gone all night and envisioned a scenario in which she somehow arose to hear a radio bulletin about the Santa Monica slasher, and if I weren't there…

In general, while lawyers invariably gird themselves to a worst-case scenario, doctors are different creatures. We survive on the hope and optimism that we can do the best for our patients: heal them, cure them, make them happy. So I gently woke my wife up, told her I was being called to duty, and sent her back to dreamland.

"Please save them, sweetheart," she said, even without having heard the grisly details. Although not a doctor herself, Karen was a partner in my practice as well as in my life. She loved medicine as much as I did for all the good it could do. She always made me want to be even better than I thought I was, and her exhortations always made me rise to the occasion, whatever it was. So I put on my coat and tie (even in emergencies, formality inspires confidence) and went off into a darkness fragrant with night-blooming jasmine and other perfumes of the paradise that had been lost to tonight's victims. It was my task to bring them back, if not to paradise, at least to life itself.

Santa Monica Hospital was about fifteen minutes away. I was on staff there, as well as many other hospitals in the Los Angeles area: Culver City, Downtown, East Los Angeles—hardly the sickrooms of the stars. My many affiliations came from my lack of any affiliations at all when I arrived in the city in 1977. Then I was truly a stranger in a strange land, a Bronx boy amidst the bougainvillea, with no friends, family, or contacts, only a burning desire to practice medicine and do surgery: have scalpel, will travel. Thus, I applied to, and was accepted by, a host of hospitals, the price of admission for which was being on call for emergencies. Although my practice had evolved beyond my wildest dreams in the two decades since my arrival, and I could have become an ivory tower Beverly Hills doctor with no bags under my eyes, I never dropped those affiliations and never stopped receiving those midnight calls. They weren't a hardship; they were a challenge. They were my life. Just as a fireman likes to put out fires, a surgeon likes to operate.

The Santa Monica Hospital Emergency Room was mobbed with policemen and reporters. Emergency rooms are rarely calm, but the one at nearby St. John's Hospital always struck me as having a greater serenity than most, perhaps because the clerical influence is more calming than the secular. A lot of Christian stars—Elizabeth Taylor, James Stewart, Henry Fonda, Michael Jackson—seemed to gravitate to St. John's rather than Cedars-Sinai (the traditional show business hospital) because of this serenity factor. It also might have had something to do with an urban myth, among doctors, that Cedars was the place where freakish accidents occurred, where bad things happened to famous people.

Danny Kaye was chairman of the board of Cedars trustees when he died from a transfusion of the wrong type blood. This kind of bizarre, theatrical only-in-Hollywood medical mishap made some people eschew the glitz associated with being taken to a place where Steven Spielberg's name is on one tower, game show king Mark Goodson's is on another, and oilman and one-time 20th Century Fox owner Marvin Davis's is on a third. Despite the towers, Goodson and Davis both died at Cedars. Tonight's victims—a highly successful television writer and his rising starlet girlfriend—had no choice in the matter. His throat was slit, her face slashed. Neither could voice a preference, and the ambulance took them to the public hospital. At the hospital, I quickly scrubbed, changed into my green surgical gown, and assessed the situation. It was bleak.

The man was gravely cut, with a large gaping wound across his entire midneck, ear to ear. He had lost a great deal of blood and was being transfused. He was conscious, however, and I introduced myself and reassured him that I would do my very best to take care of him and his girlfriend. She also was badly slashed, with an injury to the facial nerve that controlled the movement of the muscles of facial expression. But I was sure she would live. I couldn't predict whether her boyfriend would. I called two colleagues, Rod Baxter and Mark Glickman, to come assist me in what was to be a major surgical challenge.

Both doctors, as was their wont, rose to the occasion. There was no discussion of fees or insurance, just wounds and lives. Although the insurance-billing protocol of emergency room work was that an assistant surgeon received 20 percent of the main surgeon's fees, I designated Rod co-surgeon and told him I would split my fee 50-50 with him. Mark, a nerve specialist, would get the girlfriend's entire fee because she was going to be his case. Because money was not my concern, I didn't want it to be to the other doctors' either, so the easiest way to achieve maximum equity and motivation seemed to be to give it to them. The going rate at the time for the kind of throat surgery we were about to perform was around $15,000. In light of such high compensation, none of us ever thought about the money. It was there, and that was a good thing because it enabled us to focus on the main chance, which was saving or salvaging lives.

So we set off to work. What a mess! The assailant's knife had cut the trachea (windpipe), the larynx (voice box), the pharynx (throat), and the carotid artery. Rod and I were both trained as head and neck surgeons, plastic surgeons, and ear, nose, and throat specialists, and this case required all of our skills. Slowly but surely, we gained control of what had seemed, initially, like a runaway train. You're never sure at the beginning of the process what curve balls may be thrown at you, but eventually the tide begins to turn in your favor: that is the rush of surgery.

The victim's major blood vessels, trachea, and larynx all became structures to repair, and they did not seem to belong to a human being. I felt like an old world craftsman rebuilding a delicate musical instrument that had been seemingly irreparably damaged by barbaric Mongol hordes. The entire process took more than seven hours. We finished by placing a tracheostomy in our patient's windpipe (you become proprietary over the lives in your hands) so his breathing could be mechanically assisted to allow the damaged structures to heal. When we were through, I looked at the man, my man, and suddenly he was a human being again, no longer a Stradivarius or some other mechanical object, a person I had helped save. I was filled with pride, joy, and humility. Some surgeons are arrogant about being able to play God, but I knew God had a lot to do with the game of life that I was playing.

Although hardly a religious person, I was thanking God a lot those days. As I drove home with the dawn, I drank in the fragrant smells of mown grass and the glistening freshness of the morning dew. Arriving at my home, I literally stopped to smell the roses. Karen and I had developed serious green thumbs and had created our own elaborate English garden, with views all the way to the Pacific and the verdant dome of the Palos Verdes Peninsula. Some mornings we would see deer, sometimes ducks, and, on occasion, a graceful white heron would pay a visit. We figured that since we were living in paradise, we should plant our own Garden of Eden, and this was it.

Back in the house, Karen was just waking. I shared my exhilaration over the successful surgery. I would tell her the details later that day when I got to the office. I took a shower, changed into a new suit, downed an English muffin and some orange juice, and went off to make my day, and hopefully those of my patients.

For some reason, I wasn't fatigued. Medical school and the whole intern and resident process, a ten-year boot camp for doctors, had trained me to transcend sleep deprivation. Still, I couldn't help but congratulate myself on my own energy. Not bad for a guy with cancer. Not bad for a guy with maybe only a few years left to live. I tried not to think about horizons, other than the blue one of the majestic ocean out my window, but, as a doctor, I dealt in reality, and my reality was fairly bleak.

It had started in 1993 with a minor skin rash. After a grueling year-long odyssey through legions of specialists, in which the initial response went from "this is weird but nothing," to "this is weird but something" to "this is weird but fatal," I was diagnosed with a form of non-Hodgkin's lymphoma, an incurable cancer of the lymph nodes with a five-year survival rate of less than 50 percent. In other words, I had a better than average chance of being dead next year. But I wasn't dead yet. I was doing chemotherapy one week a month, and I was feeling better than I knew I had any right to: well enough to do all-night surgeries, well enough to maintain my practice, well enough to give medicine 100 percent before the law of diminishing returns set in. It may have seemed as if I was running for my life, but I had everything to live for: a wonderful wife, a wonderful career, a wonderful existence.

After my diagnosis, I went from being a lord of the medical establishment to being its vassal. It was humbling, illuminating, and terrifying to be on the other side of the desk, but the experience had made me a far better doctor. Not that I was a stranger to being on the receiving end of bad news. My father had died of stomach cancer in

1984. My mother had Parkinson's disease and had been in a nursing home for over a decade when she died in 1992. My wife's father had died of pancreatic cancer in 1989. Her mother and sister had both developed breast cancer successively in 1992 and 1993, and both had undergone mastectomies. Yet both of them were well, and I felt well, and somehow I believed that the best, not the worst, was yet to come. Although I lacked the cowboy swagger of John Wayne, in the back of my head I liked to quote the Duke's famous line, "I licked the Big C."

Of course, the irony and the tragedy was that the Duke did not, but hope may be the most powerful drug of all, and I was high on it. I lived one day at a time, and this one was shaping up to be very good. First I stopped by Cedars-Sinai, on the eastern fringe of Beverly Hills, to see a hospitalized throat cancer patient. It felt good going in as a doctor, not a patient; it felt good running into a few of my colleagues in the long corridors, being part of a community of healers, and it felt good to see my patient, a realtor in his sixties who had smoked since living in Paris on junior year abroad, wanting to be Belmondo cool, recovering so nicely from my surgery, which seemed to have gotten the entire tumor before it had spread. The cigarettes had been discarded, but he was still a Francophile. He had just started eating again, and for this his first breakfast, he was devouring a buttery *pain au chocolat*, which wouldn't have been on the menu at any other hospital but Cedars. One way the rich were different was that they ate fancier food, and as far as Cedars was concerned, *vive la différence*. In any event I was thrilled to see my patient, who was in dire straits and the depths of despair only a week before, living with such gusto. Eating well is often the best revenge.

After my hospital rounds, I drove back to Beverly Hills to the Beverwil Surgical Center, an elaborate state-of-the-art private suite of operating rooms where I performed most of my plastic surgery operations. Since I had begun practicing, Beverly Hills had replaced Rio de Janeiro as the plastic surgery capital of the world, and private surgery centers had proliferated to accommodate the enormous expansion of outpatient surgery, cosmetic as well as procedures such as endoscopies and colonoscopies that used to be performed at hospitals. These centers were a boon to patients, for they were far less expensive than the operating rooms of hospitals.

Beverwil, at the intersection of Beverly and Wilshire, was owned by a charismatic doctor named Dexter Farnham, who was not only a physical giant, a six-foot-three mountain man from Colorado, but one of the towering academic presences in the field of plastic surgery, and one of its most entrepreneurial practitioners. He had been a professor at Stanford and was now at UCLA, he lectured at Harvard, Oxford, the Sorbonne, and Tokyo University. He had an endless list of awards and publications and surgical innovations and patents, and he was considered one of the most successful physicians in a city of millionaire doctors.

Dexter operated on stars and tycoons, but he also operated on the poor. He had a chain of clinics in diverse neighborhoods: the Latino barrio of East Los Angeles, the Chinese enclave of Monterey Park, and the Little Saigon of Westminster—places where tourists seeking the glamorous LA Experience of Spago and Nobu and Mister Chow and the Polo Lounge and Rodeo Drive and Malibu would never hear of. Dexter was an evangelical plastic surgeon; he wanted to bring beauty to the masses and had the tough pioneer determination to make it happen, make people happy, and make a fortune in the process. This son of a poor cattleman was the embodiment of the American Dream, and he became such, in part, by making a new component of that dream

8

the right to look your best, and hence feel your best, no matter who you were—rich like Dexter's famous patients, or an underprivileged immigrant who watched TV and learned about the miracles of plastic surgery and wanted to be beautiful, too.

Dexter was something of a father figure to me, as well as a god. At forty-something, I was ten years his junior, and honored that he had chosen me to be part of his team and work with him at Beverwil. I had worked with great surgeons in medical school and as a resident, and now to be one of Dexter's acolytes filled me with pride and made me work that much harder. He was one of the few people I told I had cancer. His medical advice was important, and his continued professional support and insistence that I keep working—that he would never drop me from his team, whatever the circumstances—had meant the world to me. I gave Dexter a lot of the credit for my current energy and well-being. He had given me a mission to accomplish, and that mission, I felt, was keeping me alive.

That morning, I changed into surgeon's greens for the second time in twelve hours. I always felt like Clark Kent putting on the outfit, man and superman. Although the cancer had become my kryptonite, I still got a rush of invulnerability in that green scrub suit, the shoe covers, the cap, and the mask. Here I was, going off to save the world, and the change into costume somehow pumped me with the adrenaline to do so. Clothes can, and do, make the man. Suitably self-inspired, I went on to perform operations on three of Dexter's patients whom he had entrusted to me. Now they were my patients, and I treated each like a precious treasure.

First I did a rhinoplasty, or nose job, on a young Mexican hospital worker from Veracruz whose nasal septum was so deviated that she had suffered for years from a chronic sinus infection. She was living refutation of the myth that people who lived in salubrious climates, like her tropical one on the Gulf of Mexico, got fewer colds. I felt positive about her prospects for much better health. My second patient was a Chinese man, to whom I gave a chin implant. This was purely cosmetic, but the man was proof of the reality of psychosomatic illness. He had had no chin whatsoever, and no social life either. He worked as an engineer, made a good living, yet had never married, which was unusual for a Chinese male in his late thirties. He had had a rash of digestive disorders, sleep disorders, and nervous disorders. He had been worked up for brain tumors as well as for several possible malignancies, all of which turned out to be negative. He could barely meet my gaze, so ashamed of his appearance was he. Here was a prime candidate for plastic surgery. Changing his looks, I was convinced, would change his life.

My third procedure was an otoplasty, or ear reduction, on a seven-year-old French boy whose father was a major international antiques dealer. This adorable child was cursed with "Dumbo" ears, which his parents told me had made him the subject of ridicule at the elite private school he attended in Beverly Hills. All kids can be cruel, but rich kids, who socialize in a society where looks are everything and can be changed at will, can be even crueler. Despite the obviousness of the problem, I would not have operated on the boy had he not himself, and not just his parents, made it clear he wanted to make the change. "I want to look like my friends," he had said poignantly. "Can you fix me?" I was very happy to accommodate him and was glad that otoplasty was a tried and true procedure with very low risk. After the procedure, when he awoke, his head wrapped and bandaged, he took a long time to react. I had no idea what that reaction would be. I was much more anxious about his psychological response to the surgery than his physical one. When he finally said, "The mummy—c'est cool," and broke into a weak smile, I couldn't have been more relieved.

I washed up, got back into my suit, thanked the anesthesiologist, the nurses, and the office staff at Beverwil, and made sure my three patients were recovering well and would be discharged on schedule that day. Then I drove to my office on Roxbury Drive. This street, along with Bedford Drive, constitutes the Beverly Hills equivalent of London's Harley Street, the famous boulevard of the golden scalpel, where all the great British surgeons (who, in a very British display of reverse-snob nomenclature, were called *Mister* rather than *Doctor*) were located. My area was known as the Golden Triangle, for it was encompassed by a geometry of streets bounded by Wilshire and Santa Monica Boulevards. It might also have been called the Plastic Triangle, for the many top plastic surgeons who had their offices there.

Beverly Hills plastic surgeon. That's what I was, and to everyone I ever met, it sounded incredibly cool, the apotheosis of medical practice. The image was that of doctor to the stars, living in the most fabled town on earth, making tons of money, operating on celebrities, doing breast implants on Demi Moore and liposuction on Elizabeth Taylor and facelifts on Robert Redford, or going to Lakers games with Jack Nicholson and his cardiologist, or to the Playboy Mansion with Hef's urologist, or to the golf course at the Riviera Country Club with Jerry Seinfeld's psychiatrist, and wherever you went, it was always in a Mercedes.

Well, the Mercedes part was true, and as I pulled into my reserved space in my building's parking structure, it was as if I had made a turn into a Mercedes dealership rather than into a medical building. There were so many fancy cars that I was reminded of the fabled parking area of Ma Maison restaurant (so exclusive its phone number was unlisted) where the valets would line up the guests' vehicles out front according to the status of the cars: Ferraris, then Bentleys, then Rollses, with Mercedes relegated to the back rows (except for collectors' Gullwings), and BMWs parked in a hidden auxiliary lot across the street.

So I had a Mercedes, and my wife did, too, but for us, these cars were simply reliable transportation, not a show of force. And, yes, we lived in exclusive Bel Air in a seven-figure house, and I earned a seven-figure income, and I did treat movie stars and rock stars and top models and Fortune 500 types. But so did thirty or forty other Beverly Hills plastic surgeons, and most of the people we treated were ordinary folks, just like us. It was actually a tiny community, but it was my community, and I wasn't at all impressed by it until out-of-town friends came and drooled over how fantastic it all seemed.

All of us had our share of glamour and success, but this was where I worked, and I took the money and the glamour for granted. What mattered to me were the patients, no matter who they were, and the medical and surgical challenges they presented. I had money, and I had glamour, but I also had cancer. I knew full well what my priorities were.

On my way up to my office, I ran into one of the real "doctors to the stars," Rex Kennamer, whose office was down the hall from mine. Then in his eighties, Rex was tall, white-haired, and theatrically distinguished, with a great resonant, accentless voice that inspired confidence. It was said that Rex was the inspiration for the comic strip *Rex Morgan, M.D.*, but he would never own up to it, just as he would never brag about who his patients were. But everybody knew that the really big stars of the forties and fifties— before "the pictures got small," as Gloria Swanson put it in *Sunset Boulevard*—were Kennamer patients: Bogart, Cagney, Ladd, Crawford, Davis, Taylor.

Karen's mother, Mimi, a great beauty who had been the private secretary to producer Jack Warner in Hollywood's glory days, knew all the gossip: who treated whom, who slept with whom, who killed whom. Sometimes you'd see the aging legends limping or being wheeled into Rex's office, and it reminded you just how ephemeral the beauty and the glitter really were. Now, years later, Rex still showed up every day. Like old soldiers who never died, old doctors were destined to fade away. I prayed I would be so lucky.

The other famous doctors to the stars who were still alive—either in body or in the town's imagination—when I started practice in 1977 had by now faded completely. There was Red Krohn, Frank Sinatra's doctor, who was also known as the celebrity abortionist in the Eisenhower era. There was Ralph Greenson, Marilyn Monroe's psychiatrist, whose wife was the sister of Sinatra's all-powerful lawyer, Mickey Rudin. And there was Hy Engelberg, Marilyn's internist, whose son Michael became an oncologist and treated many of the celebrities he inherited from his father. Such was the web of family ties and interlocking relationships that had allowed a very few doctors to gain a medical monopoly on the closed shop that was Hollywood back when the studios controlled the stars and Beverly Hills was basically a small town where everyone happened to be rich.

With the rise of television, there were a lot more stars, and a lot more doctors. By the mid-90s, there was a vast amount of plastic surgery, which had become the most booming field of medicine, at least in these rarefied climes. This was a decade before the rise of the plastic surgery reality shows like *Extreme Makeover* or dramatic fare like *Doctor 90210* and *Nip Tuck*. Now plastic surgeons have film agents, press agents, media coaches, Web sites, and DVDs. Their names are well known because so many people are watching them on the small screen. But in the mid-90s, the only publicity most plastic surgeons enjoyed was an ad they paid for in the back of *Los Angeles Magazine*. Ads pitched to the public always seemed embarrassingly unprofessional to me, and I steadfastly refused to do it.

The one plastic surgeon who had some public notoriety was a colleague named Harry Glassman; he had been married to *Dallas* star Victoria Principal. Celebrity clients were pretty well spread out among the plastic surgeons of Beverly Hills. Client referrals happened almost randomly. You would treat an accountant who happened to be the trusted CPA of some movie star whom the accountant would send to you. Once you had done a good job, the star would recommend you to other stars, or maybe to other CPAs, depending on the star's circle of friends.

The plastic surgeon best known for treating stars was Steve Hoefflin, a very unglamorous burn specialist who had treated Michael Jackson when the singer caught fire and was taken to the Brotman Burn Center in Culver City. Jackson loved what Steve did and then recommended him to his best friend Elizabeth Taylor. From then on, the tabloids were camped outside Steve's Santa Monica offices and a glittering reputation was born—this even though Michael Jackson was not the best poster boy for plastic surgery.

It is true that a star's endorsement can seem to the public like the Good Housekeeping Seal of Approval, or the equivalent of the British label "By Appointment to Her Majesty," and some doctors, not just plastic surgeons, thrive on it. One dermatologist, Arnie Klein, nicknamed "King Collagen" because of his pioneering work with the substance, sought and courted stars, and usually had a line of limos clogging the street in front of his office, a block away from mine. Klein was the recently acquitted defendant in the Irena Medavoy (wife of a studio head) Botox litigation, in which Medavoy unsuccessfully alleged that Klein's work caused her crippling migraines as well as more serious maladies. But the pursuit of beauty is hard to deter, and Klein's Bedford Street practice seemed only to have profited from all the publicity.

The doctor in the area with the most stars as patients wasn't a plastic surgeon but a "natural healer" on Bedford named Saram Khalsa, who was actually a nice Jewish boy from Cleveland and a Case Western Reserve MD who had become a Sikh sometime during his post-college years and donned a turban and flowing white robes. His specialty was yeast infections. He put people on the most restrictive diets imaginable and prescribed exorbitantly expensive vitamins and herbs out of his Taj Mahalian offices. The stars, especially the young female supernovas, came in droves.

There were no stars in my office that day, just ordinary people with real concerns, some valid, some not. My office, at 436 Roxbury, was in a two-story red brick building that was built just before World War II. There was nothing particularly glamorous about it, except that it was pure Hollywood, full of every kind of specialist who had treated every star from Astaire to Zadora. The place had a film noir feel in a Raymond Chandler sort of way and that was its charm. The halls had plush, deep green carpets, and the doors were thick oak with shiny brass handles. I had tried to keep the look of my office the same as when I had taken it over in 1978. None of my predecessors had wanted to change it, either, so I guess I'd describe the style as prewar Palm Springs: blond wood paneling, patio-style furnishings, bean-pole standing lamps, prints of birds and flowers and California deserts and mountains. Some rooms had banana-leaf wallpaper, similar to the famous wall coverings of the Polo Lounge at the Beverly Hills Hotel.

None of our furnishings were original. Karen and I had scoured the souks and galleries of Southern California to create the effect. The decorating was great fun. Because Karen and I were gardeners, we had a fabulous profusion of plants and flowers from our home, of which this office was a natural extension. Karen had also added a fish tank, which to me was more Dr. No than Dr. Reiter, but its effect was to keep the patients calm. There were countless magazines, from *The New Yorker* to *Vogue* to *Sports Illustrated*; whatever we had would inevitably be stolen by the patients, but that was one of the costs of doing business. The mood was truly California retro, and I hoped that the effect would put my patients in a retro mood, reminding them of times that were not so competitive or stressful.

I was greeted by my cheerful receptionist, Caroline, my loyal nurse, Josie, and then by Karen, who basically served as my office manager and source of all that was sane and sensible. She had brought me a tuna salad from Walter's on Canon Drive, which was reputed to be the best tuna salad in the world by coffee shop gourmets—a tuna salad that, were it less perishable, might have been shipped by agents to film shoots around the world the way Chasen's chili was sent to Rome to Elizabeth Taylor when she made the epic fiasco *Cleopatra*. Karen knew I needed nutrition, and that unless she got it for me, I would forget about it. Doctors can run on empty, but doctors with cancer shouldn't, and Karen took on the role of nurse-nutritionist to a person who twelve-steppers might say was in denial.

Sitting at my office desk, whose avalanche of papers Karen had transformed into ordered sculpture, I wolfed down the tart and creamy tuna and brought Karen up to date on my morning's triumphs. She seemed almost as excited as I was, but then tried to get me to focus on the more quotidian matters of running the office, which, much as I ignored the idea, had to be treated as a business. All surgeons see themselves as artists, and all artists hate paperwork. I much preferred to leave the paperwork to her. I had people to take care of. People, with me, always came first. Karen gave me a knowing shrug and a loving kiss on the cheek and let me do my thing.

My first patient was an African American woman in her early thirties on whom I had done a rhinoplasty with, I thought, great results. I wish she had been half as happy, but she was suffering a surgical variation of buyer's remorse. She wanted to be twice as happy, and unrealistically so. Her "new" nose had made her start rethinking her entire face. She now wanted chin work, eye work, cheek work. The woman was a model, once a fashion and runway near-star, now a frequent face on television commercials. She had decided she didn't like her nose, that it was too broad and didn't fit her otherwise delicate facial features. So, after much going back and forth, having considered countless noses from classical sculpture to Harper's Bazaar, we decided to proceed. Now she was completely healed; the swelling and bruising were gone, the new look in place. And instead of being content, she was more unsatisfied than before. "My nose is so great, but what about the rest of me?" she despaired.

She was more beautiful than ever, I assured her.

"The nose is too good. Let's bring the rest up to speed. Otherwise that nose is going to stand out as fake," she pleaded. "My face is my moneymaker. Come on, Dr. Reiter. Please…"

Being a plastic surgeon involves also being a psychologist, or psychiatrist, to whom I would invariably have to refer some patients - those seeking to transform themselves into something they could never be. Plastic surgery can raise your self-esteem, to be sure, but it was never

17

intended as a panacea. In this patient's case, I tried to explain to her how fine she looked, and how further attempts to push the envelope of her beauty could end disastrously. "Perfection is never perfect. But you're pretty close. You fly too close to the sun, you could melt," I told her, invoking Icarus. She gave me a blank stare. Sometimes I forgot I was in Los Angeles, where classical references tend not to play. I wished I had watched more television, to get some more accessible analogies, but who had the time? "You're a beautiful woman," I told her, "a beautiful woman who earns a wonderful living from her beauty."

"But I want to earn more!" she said.

"Don't be greedy," I tried to joke with her. "Don't look a gift horse in the nose."

She laughed, but I'm not sure if I would have won the day if it hadn't been for Karen, who dropped in, unprompted, and exclaimed, "Oh, my God. I love it! You look so great! A young Diana Ross. I never saw that before." Karen, who had helped prep this woman for surgery and all its aftermath, had not seen her for more than a month. Karen was unable to fake sincerity; anyone who knew her could see this. Halle Berry wasn't yet a star, and Diana Ross was *le mot just*, as the French would say. This was plastic surgery, Hollywood-style, and you had to be able to talk the talk. But you had to listen as well. This patient was hell-bent on maximizing her beauty. My job was to keep her from going overboard. Eventually, after many discussions, we settled on putting a dimple in her chin and doing her eyelids, and then stopping while we were way ahead. A few years later, this patient won the Mrs. California Pageant and nearly won Mrs. America. I couldn't have been prouder of her, or my work.

My next patient was a prim, fortyish schoolteacher from the elite Harvard-Westlake School in Beverly Hills who saw herself as the least likely candidate in the world for plastic surgery. She was in my office to convince herself to shed her stereotypical inhibitions that the only people who underwent cosmetic procedures were "plastic" media stars and superficial Valley girls. She didn't want to be Pamela Anderson. She wanted to be Jane Fonda. I happened to know that Jane Fonda had recently had breast implants, so the notion of the classy "natural" celebrity was out the window.

Still, the teacher needed more convincing. We embarked upon a cat-and-mouse game, in which she tried to get me to tell her what she *needed* and I tried to get her to tell me what she *wanted*. Eventually, she conceded that she hated what was happening to her eyes. In plastic surgeon parlance, she was in the first stage of considering a blepharoplasty, or eyelid surgery, an excision of excess skin on her upper eyelid and the removal of orbital fat, which was causing bags under her eyes. "I used to think it gave me a scholarly look," she told me, "but now I think I'm just turning into an old bag."

After assuring her of her own attractiveness and of the "respectability" of the procedure, I explained how dramatic a difference this relatively simple operation could make. If anything in cosmetic surgery could turn back the clock, it is eye work. I had performed many such procedures on the mothers of many of her students, as well as on starlets from the Playboy Mansion, a block from her school. I do believe I won her over, though, by a discourse into the history of the procedure, which respected her obvious intelligence as well as played to it. I did my etymological bit, explaining the Greek origin of the name of the procedure, "blepharos" meaning the eye, "plastos" to form. The Roman encyclopedist Aulus Cornelius Celsus, who lived and worked from 25 B.C. to 50 A.D. had written about eyelid procedures.. The great Arab surgeon Ali ben Isa in the ninth century, described a procedure in which the excessive folds of aging eyelid skin were held between two tightened wooden mini-bars for ten days until the skin, deprived of nutrition, died and fell off, leaving no scar.

Today the procedure has evolved from what sounded like medieval torture into a minimally painless state-of-the-art outpatient surgery. I loved doing blepharoplasties, which are among the most elegant of all plastic surgery procedures. The anatomy of the eyelid is unparalleled in delicacy, detail, and function, and it is a measure of the surgeon's skill how well eyelid surgery turns out; with something so intricate, lots can go wrong. The challenge of each operation never ceased to inspire me. The eyes, in my opinion, are the prime contributor to the expressiveness of the face. The aging process diminishes this expressiveness. The bags of the lower lids are symbols of fatigue, and it was always an exhilarating opportunity for me to remove the bulging fat that causes these bags either by an incision in the skin itself, or behind the skin, in the conjunctiva, or inner lining of the eye. It may sound grisly, but it isn't, really, and compared to what the Arabs did ten centuries ago, it's a picnic for the patient. In the end, the patient always looked much younger, and I would feel like a magician.

After about an hour of my own pedagogy (a wall of books behind me didn't hurt as backup), the teacher felt she had learned her lesson and was ready to cross the Rubicon. I took her into our photo room and took "before" photographs with my Minolta camera. This was just before the advent of razzle-dazzle computer imaging, and I felt like an old-fashioned Matthew Brady setting up the umbrella flash against the light blue screen that had been installed by the wizards of Sammy's Cameras, the top photographic outfit in the city. I could have delegated this work to the nurse or hired a tech for the job, but I liked to do it myself to show the patients that I was involved with them every step of the way.

Karen was the true "closer" in any new patient situation, though pressure salesmanship was the furthest thing from her nature. She simply radiated wholesomeness, good taste, sincerity, and, above all, caring. After I finished my consultation with a patient, Karen would take her into her office and reiterate all the details of her surgery, including the costs, insurance coverage, what to expect in terms of preparation and recovery, what drugs to discontinue, everything. I used to scold Karen, saying she'd scare the patients away because she'd go over every worst-case scenario, but she was a worst-case kind of girl and I often teased that she should have been a lawyer. To my surprise, the patients appreciated her full disclosure, all the more so when she also told them how great she thought they'd look after their surgery.

Aside from a few minor skin procedures, Karen had never had any surgery, never wanted any, never needed any. She had a perfect nose, perfect skin, and huge, dazzling green eyes. Her most unforgettable feature were those eyes, flirtatious, vivacious eyes that could get you 'in a whole lot of trouble' as 'Them There Eyes,' the old Billie Holiday blues song, went. Yet Karen wasn't interested in trouble, in playing the femme fatale. She was way too kind for that. Karen's Achilles heel, since her teen years, had been her weight, and every meal was a war with temptation (she loved great food) to keep her sleek figure. But the patients only saw the end product of all her self-control battles, and Karen's fine looks and matching character inspired confidence. I may have 'made' the faces, but Karen made my business. Notwithstanding my cluelessness about, and general disinterest in money, Karen's charm and energy had made me, at least on paper, a rich man. 'Beverly Hills Doctor' is a cliché the world may envy, but it was one both Karen and I strove to transcend by living for our patients and not ourselves.

My next patient was a young lawyer in his twenties who was just starting his career and wanted a fresh start with a straight nose instead of his large, crooked one, a nose that had accentuated his narrow, thin face. Unlike local female patients, who flocked to nasal stereotypes, particularly the perky all-American Meg Ryan model, the males didn't want to look like anyone in particular; they just wanted to look good. This was before Adrian Brody's Oscar for *The Pianist* made hooked noses chic.

Today was the unveiling of the hopeful masterpiece I had created the week before, the removal of the bandages. As a preamble, I asked the patient if he had had any troubles, such as nosebleeds, infections, discharge, all of which can happen, even in the most successful operations. He said no, impatiently. All he cared about was the main event. His old nose had an angle between its tip and the upper lip that was less than ninety degrees, which plastic surgeons label as "acute." The result was the impression that his face was in a sad, downward direction, a no-no in our upbeat times. I had removed bone and cartilage to straighten his profile and raise the tip of his nose. To improve his breathing, I corrected his septum to equalize his air passages. Now we would see what it looked like.

I'm always nervous in these situations because, no matter how many nose jobs you've done, every patient is different, and you never know how anyone will react. With Karen looking on, always more confident and certain than I could ever be, I cut away the plaster cast and tape from the lawyer's nose. The nurse came in to clean up the sticky tape residue from the skin and spruce things up. Then I handed the young man the mirror. The moment of truth was upon us. I said nothing, as I had learned never to jump the gun and react before the patient responded. In this case it seemed to take an eternity. Then his face lit up. He was beaming. He got up and hugged me, then Karen, thanking us profusely. "You changed my life!" he exclaimed.

"No one's seen it yet," I said, not wanting to rain on his parade, but always erring on the side of caution.

"Oh, they will, Dr. Reiter, they will!"

Here a nose, and not clothes, had made the man.

My next patient was as miserable as the young lawyer was happy. She was a thirty-something real estate agent who had come to Beverly Hills from a small town in Georgia and wanted all the glamour attendant to her relocation. Part of the Beverly Hills package, for her, meant a nose job. It wasn't as if she hadn't needed it, or I would have surely turned her away, referring her to another plastic surgeon—I had plenty of colleagues who had no problem acceding to unrealistic wishes. This young woman had a bump on the dorsum, or upper surface of the nose, with a wide tip and a slightly hanging columella, the division between the two nostrils. The result was that the angle between the nose and the upper lip was also acute in her case, as it had been in the lawyer's, less than ninety degrees. In women, the standard of beauty, at least as determined over the years by surgeons, is 105 degrees from the vertical.

I had given her precisely that, and she had been thrilled at first. She claimed she was selling more condos, being pursued by more lawyers, doctors, and film agents, and was loving her Beverly Hills life. But now, nine months after the surgery (I have my patients come in about six times in the first year, which is how long it takes a rhinoplasty to heal completely), she was in a major funk. She unsheathed a

Premiere magazine, opened it to a full-page picture of Winona Ryder, and slammed it on my desk. "This is what we should have done," she declared angrily.

It's always awful when a patient is dissatisfied. I subscribed to the old adage that the customer is always right. But how could I have read this woman's mind? Winona Ryder had never entered any of our discussions. I noticed now that the woman had dyed her light brown hair black and cut it as well, obviously in an attempt to replicate Winona's gamine appearance. And the nose didn't fit.

"I'm not glamorous enough," she said, despairing. She was a small-town Southern girl who had moved to the land of the stars seeking the glamour she had heard about all her life. Part of the Beverly Hills experience, she had concluded, was looking like a movie star, something she had never mentioned to me before. I was so pleased with her nose; it fit her face perfectly and was an excellent cosmetic result. Unfortunately, many people have a preconceived notion as to how their new appearance can change their lives. It's one thing to fantasize about stars, or sports heroes, or even Internet moguls, but it takes more than an altered nose to alter your life. This patient needed more than confidence, which this beautiful new nose should have given her. She wanted a lifestyle change, which is out of the realm of the surgeon. A guru might have helped.

All my reassurances fell on deaf ears. I praised the balance of her nose, the symmetry of it with the rest of her face, the classical angles between her nose and forehead and between her nose and her upper lip, and its new aquiline straightness. Nothing mattered. It wasn't Winona. Karen, whom I called in for help, had a different approach. She assured the patient that she was prettier than Winona, and enumerated detail after detail to make the case. It didn't work. The woman wanted new surgery, and she wanted it for free, as if the doctor is a guarantor of the desired result, even if that desire is as slippery as mercury. The best that I could do was to ask her to think it over for a month. I prayed she would changer her mind once again.

It was nearly five o'clock, the end of a long day, but there were several patients left to see. It always took longer than we scheduled because people need lots of attention, especially where looks are concerned. My next patient was a handsome, strong-jawed man in his mid-thirties, tall and rugged, with the Marlboro name of Clint Marlin. He was accompanied by a statuesque blonde of about the same age. I couldn't understand why either of them would be in a plastic surgeon's office. On his patient information sheet, the man didn't specify why he had come. The woman spoke with a foreign accent. She introduced herself as Sigrid Brunner. She told me she was from Colombia, and my initial, unfair thought was that she was the grandchild of some flight Nazi who escaped to South America to avoid the Nuremberg Trials.

"Could you please close the door?" Sigrid asked me.

The office had old-fashioned sliding doors that were difficult to close. I always left them open. "It's very private," I assured them. "No one can overhear us."

"It's better if you close the door, Dr. Reiter," Clint insisted in a deeply authoritative voice. I looked closely at him. Did he need a hair transplant? What procedure that I might do could be that embarrassing to him? I got up to close the door. It squeaked terribly and made such a racket that Karen came out to see if something was wrong.

"Ve vant to be alone," I made a Greta Garbo joke and then worried that Sigrid might think I was making fun of her accent.

I sat back down at my desk. Before I could ask them what I could do for them, each of them stood up and flashed a badge at me. Then they reintroduced themselves as FBI agents.

The last time law enforcement had entered my office was in 1980, when the Beverly Hills Police Department showed up to investigate one of my ENT patients, a nice old lady in her seventies who used to bring me gifts of rare wines, like Chateau Lafitte Rothschild or Chateau d'Yquem. I had no idea just how rare they were until I brought them as house gifts to dinner parties and my hosts would nearly faint at my generosity. It turned out that the lady was shoplifting the wines from all the fancy wine stores in the neighborhood, and the police had arrested her. I covered for her, denying she had ever given me any presents. At her age, she didn't need to be taught any more lessons, much less go to jail.

So now my first thought was that the FBI must be investigating one of my patients, a secret criminal perhaps who had a facelift to change his identity and outwit the law. As I racked my mind to figure out who among my patients could be so daringly imaginative, Sigrid cut off that line of thought. "We're investigating the Beverwil Surgery Center, Dr. Reiter. We'd like you to tell us all you know about it."

I had no idea what they were after, but I wasn't about to say anything about my friend and mentor Dexter Farnham. He had stood by me in my darkest hour, had given me a continued lease on life, and, besides, he was one of the finest men in our field. Maybe someone else there had done something wrong, another doctor perhaps, an employee, an unexplained death, somebody smuggling cocaine. My mind raced but came up blank.

"We know you've been sick, Dr. Reiter," Clint, or rather Special Agent Marlin, said ominously. "Actually, you look pretty good. I'd never know you had anything," he added even more ominously, totally invading my privacy. Outside of Karen, Dexter, and my doctors, no one knew I was sick. News of my condition would be fatal to my practice. "But there are well-founded allegations of some very serious criminal activity at the center," he went on. "You know what we're talking about."

"No, I don't. I'm sorry." I said.

"This kind of thing is happening everywhere. We're talking millions of dollars here and nationwide," Marlin added.

I still had no inkling of what they were talking about that could be the stuff of gangbusters. The big crime issue in medicine at that time was Medicare and Medicaid fraud, which apparently was up in the billions of dollars, usually involving huge health care outfits cooking their books and falsifying claims reports. There seemed to be a new atrocity of this sort reported every week in the Wall Street Journal, but it was all so confusing only a few CPAs could possibly understand it. Perhaps that was how these huge outfits had been getting away with it, by boring the regulators to death.

But the Beverwil Surgery Center? And that pillar of rectitude Dexter Farnham? Dexter was a genius, in surgery, in math, in everything. When I had gotten sick, Dexter insisted on taking over my billing, knowing how soul crushing I found the business part. I felt he was doing me a favor.

A lot of doctors distrusted insurance companies and held them accountable for many of the ills in modern medicine. No one disliked them more than the Colorado populist, the mountain man of rugged individuality, Dexter Farnham. He believed that everyone should have a shot at plastic surgery, if it would make his or her life better— whoever was poor and struggling and wanted to look better and feel better.

Dexter was one of the most successful and richest doctors in LA. That had probably made him a target. "I love the center. They do great work. Dexter Farnham's a giant. He's a wonderful man. I really have nothing else to say," I said.

Sigrid nearly rolled her eyes in disgust. She exchanged looks with Clint. "Do you have a lawyer, Dr. Reiter?" she asked me.

"Of course not," I replied, maybe too emphatically. "I don't really need one."

"You need one now," she snapped, and presented me with a subpoena to appear before the grand jury in several weeks.

"You have enough trouble, Dr. Reiter," Sigrid said, all vicious threat. "It's bad enough to be sick. It's a lot worse to be sick in prison for what's left of your life. Have a nice day."

The two agents stood up, powered the sliding door open with the most awful screech, and were gone. Karen rushed in. She hadn't seen me look so pale since I received my cancer diagnosis. I was speechless. I did know one thing. Sigrid had to have Nazi genes in her somewhere.

Chapter Two

BRONX SCIENCE

One of the reasons Dexter Farnham had made such a huge impression on me was that he was the sort of character I would never have met in the Bronx, where I grew up. Dexter had truly strong character, absolute self-confidence, and a total lack of low self-esteem, which I always called the Bronx birth defect. It's hard for outsiders to imagine such successes as Bronxites Ralph Lauren and Calvin Klein as men with self-esteem issues, but it's not hard for me. Most of my classmates at the esteemed Bronx High School of Science were plagued with the curse of our parents' immigrant/Depression mentality, not to mention the second-classness of growing up in the shadow of Manhattan. This was as true for those who became professors, judges, and tycoons as it was for those who went on to win Nobel Prizes.

In my boyhood in the fifties and sixties, the borough was an upwardly mobile paradise of art deco apartment buildings and magnificent tree-shaded boulevards such as the Grand Concourse, which my parents proudly bragged was wider than Paris' Champs Elysees. Not that my parents had ever been to Paris. Their idea of a holiday was to go out to the beach at Far Rockaway, or up to the Catskills. That I would end up in California, in Beverly Hills where the stars lived, and a surgeon, a plastic surgeon, would have sounded to them like science fiction.

Like most people in the Bronx, whether Jewish, Irish, or Italian, my folks were happy just to be there, and not in the tenements and sweatshops of the Lower East Side, which had looked comparatively wonderful to their parents, glad to escape pogroms or wars or famines. It was all relative. But we knew we weren't in Manhattan, which was the Big Time. New York in those days was dominated by old-guard WASPs and old-guard German Jews—Astors, Vanderbilts, Lehmans, Warburgs—who had made their fortunes before, during, and just after the Civil War, while our forbears were serfs under the tsars. Although, as young men we hoped to amount to something someday, we always knew our place, and we always knew we weren't the ruling class. We knew we were squarely in the middle, and lucky for it.

My childhood dream was to become an engineer and build bridges in Brazil, a dream that must have come from the National Geographic, for that magazine, and the Bronx Zoo, were as close to a jungle as I would ever get. I had no interest in medicine. My first memory of a hospital was the Royal Hospital on the Grand Concourse, where I was born, and where I went with tonsillitis when I was four. I remember being in a big bed, and I remember a great feeling of relief when for some reason the doctors called off the tonsillectomy and gave me a reprieve. I had been all alone in that white room, crying to go home, and I got my wish. My tonsils eventually shrank, and I never had to undergo that dreaded surgery, which hovered over my early years like the grim reaper with a scythe. It was ironic that I would go on to become that grim reaper, an ENT specialist. Otherwise, I was a very sickly kid. I had asthma, scarlet fever, bronchitis, you name it. My mother, Pearl, a housewife, doted on me. My father, Eli, wasn't around that much. He was a manufacturer of ladies' coats, with an office at

30

the corner of Seventh Avenue and 40th Street in the garment district, to which he took the D train every day. He usually came home after I was asleep.

Whenever I was sick, which was often, my mother would bundle me up and take me to a towering limestone flatiron building on the Grand Concourse known as the Medical Arts Building. This was the Bronx's answer to Harley Street, where all its top doctors were located, but to a young kid, the term "medical arts" smacked of witchcraft and black magic. There was not one doctor my mother took me to whom I vaguely liked. One of them gave me shots inside my nose to control allergies. Talk about medieval torture. Maybe subconsciously I later went into the ENT field to bring humanity to a field that to me was all sadomasochism. So much did I dread those visits to the flatiron of painful injections and foul-tasting medicine that by the time I was twelve, I decided to change my fate. I began reading *Muscle Beach Magazine*, lifting weights, eating carrots, and drinking skim milk. No ninety-seven-pound weakling was I going to be! I began playing stickball at the nearby schoolyard and running junior high track in Van Cortlandt Park, which I reached by subway. It may seem odd to take the underground to exercise and fresh air, but such was life in New York.

I was always a good student. Being sick in my room left me little to do except study and maybe take a break to watch the *Gillette Friday Night Fights* with my father. My mother wanted me to become a schoolteacher, and took me on excursions to the local public library so that she could help me carry back all the books she inspired me to read. I skipped the eighth grade and got high scores on the exam that got me admitted to the Bronx High School of Science, which was to ambitious Jews what Exeter and Andover were to the American Establishment.

31

Bronx High may have been the most competitive, cutthroat school on earth. I wish it had taught me to be ruthless, but all it did was make me want to withdraw from the academic fray. I ended up near the top of the bottom half of my class. Content to be a small fish in a big pond, I blissfully ran track and field and studied at my own pace. I would let the career chips fall where they may.

I had shared a bedroom in our deco apartment on Mount Hope Place with my older brother, Ira, until he finished Taft High School with less than flying colors and moved to Manhattan to seek his fortune. Ira was a handsome ladies' man who resembled a young John Derek, the Svengali behind Bo and Linda Evans and other look-alike California blondes. Ira was a fast talker. My parents called him "the lover." I was "the scholar." Ira's first job was as an assistant to the head window dresser at Macy's. In later times, I would have assumed that would have made him gay (I had no idea what gay was then), but it didn't and he wasn't. He thought his job was a good way to meet beautiful women, and it was. Once he left home, Ira rarely came back, which was fine with me, since I got the bedroom all to myself. I could stay up late and study to Cousin Brucie on WABC playing all those great Elvis and Drifters and Platters and indigenous New York do-wop songs of the late '50s and early '60s. Throughout high school I never had a girlfriend, which didn't make me gay, either, but was pretty much par for the course in the temple of nerdity I attended.

My father, like Ira, and unlike me, was a ladies' man in a ladies' business, as I would learned as when I got older. I guess temptation was an occupational hazard in the garment district. My father had grown up on Orchard Street on the Lower East Side, in an Italian enclave. His best friend, and my godfather, was a gangster named Johnny Dio, and he had friends with names like "Three Finger Larry" and "Fat Tony" who were in the Teamsters or the Mob, or both. I was surprised that with these contacts my father was always struggling in his business. His Jewish friends were building big national brands, like Bobbie Brooks and Evan-Picone, while my father was constantly taking loans and renaming his line. Once, when Ira got himself in major hot water with some strong-arm bookies, our father called on Johnny Dio to bail him out.

Although I had thought I had put my childhood maladies behind me, I could never seem to get away from illness and infirmity. My father's mother, Celia, lived with us. She was a wonderful woman who read to me and gave me my love of books. She was also a great cook, which my mother was not, making all the classic Jewish dishes like pot roast and latkes and gefilte fish and pierogies that my father joked "killed more Jews than Hitler." She spoke to my parents in Yiddish, which I first thought was to keep secrets from me. I knew Celia loved me too much to do anything bad to me. At some stage she began forgetting things, then she started defecating on the floor, and then my parents put her into a nursing home. She died soon afterward. I guess she had Alzheimer's, but no one told me. Hers was my first funeral, in a Hebrew cemetery in the Bronx. I hated it. I missed my grandma, was troubled deeply by her sudden vulnerability. And then she was gone forever. I remember being very sad and crying and hoping something like that would never happen again.

In my athletic transformation, I had joined the Boy Scouts. In the summer when I was fifteen, I took a bicycle trip with my troop along the Hudson River to Dobbs Ferry. Swerving to avoid a pedestrian, I flipped my bike over a large pipe and went flying into the air, crashing to the ground into a shallow pool of water. Because I was knocked unconscious, those three or so inches of water nearly drowned me. I was rushed to a local hospital, where I remained in a coma for three days. I recovered, but my mother was worried and took me to a Park Avenue neurosurgeon for a further examination, to be sure I had no damage to my brain or nervous system. This man seemed different from the Medical Arts doctors: colder, grander. His offices were certainly far nicer, with lots of diplomas from Harvard and Yale and Massachusetts General Hospital on the walls of the leathery, clubby room. He seemed patrician and unfriendly, as if we were poor Cossacks who had invaded his rarefied domain. In any event, he gave me a quick once-over and showed us out, in a kind of bum's rush.

Mother should have been relieved, but she wasn't. Within a year, she was diagnosed with Parkinson's disease, and she blamed it on the scare my injury had given her. It started with a small tremor and gradually got worse. My father stepped up to the responsibility of her increasing care, both at home and for the frequent trips to the Albert Einstein Medical Center, but I could see that it aged him rapidly. I remember watching him in the room with my mother, staring silently out the window. He wanted to go out and live his life, but now his life was increasingly wrapped up in her care and his duty to her. I realized then that all of us have our own chains, visible and invisible.

It never occurred to me to become a doctor, to develop a cure for my beloved mother. I assumed the medical arts, such as they were, were way beyond me. Anyway, I had decided I wanted to go to West Point. I had visited the military academy on another Boy Scout excursion and thought it was the most impressive place I could dream of. Inspired, I began reading about its graduates, from Robert E. Lee to Douglas MacArthur to George Patton to the football hero Pete Dawkins. I decided that instead of being a typical Bronx Science bookworm, I would become a general, a decisive leader, a man of action, a man like the Dexter Farnham I would meet decades later.

My mother, it turned out, had Mob connections, too, just as good as my father's. Her best childhood friend, Chippy, was now the long-term mistress of an Italian mobster named Frankie Brown who controlled the numbers racket in Harlem. Our Bronx congressman was reputed to be in Frankie's pocket. He had gotten Chippy's son into Harvard Law School. I thus got the brilliant idea that Mother should call in a chip with Chippy to get Frankie to lean hard on the congressman to get me an appointment to West Point. My mother was appalled, not at the idea of the big fix but at the notion of my going up the Hudson. "No Jewish boy should go to West Point," she shrieked. So much for the Army.

Instead I headed for engineering school. Maybe I'd build those bridges in Brazil after all. Although I had high SATs and won a New York State Regents Scholarship that would have enabled me to go to Cornell, because of my mother's illness I wanted to stay at home and be near her. So I enrolled in The City College of New York, which was the total opposite of West Point but a natural extension of Bronx Science. City College had a beautiful Gothic campus that unfortunately was on Convent Avenue in the middle of Harlem. I'd take the subway there and back every morning and evening, hopefully not too late, as in those crime and graffiti-filled days, riding the subway was a harrowing experience, especially in the heart of darkness that was the City College neighborhood. I kept my nose in my books so as not to attract attention.

After two years and excellent grades, I was able to transfer to Columbia's School of Engineering. Columbia's majestic Morningside Heights campus was adjacent to Harlem but not in it. It thus felt significantly safer. Moreover, Columbia was New York's premier university. It was Ivy League. It had centuries of prestige. I was honored to be there, even as an aspiring engineer, as opposed to a future literature professor like Columbia's great Lionel Trilling or an eminent historian like the legendary Richard Hofstadter. I was able to cross register in those great men's courses, and they inspired me not to become an engineer.

Engineering was too technical, but I wasn't literary enough to consider a career in academe. Besides, academe was often for brilliant rich kids who could afford to live on a teacher's low salary. I needed a real profession, which for me became a choice between law or medicine, which wasn't much choice at all. I didn't see myself as Albert Schweitzer or Christian Barnard or any other savior of mankind. I had good grades, I was in a great school, and I needed a future. So I enrolled in all the pre-med courses: organic chemistry, biology, all the stuff that Bronx Science had well prepared me for. And I spent the next two years, not at Ivy League football games or fraternity parties, or going to Broadway shows or the Met or Carnegie Hall like so many of Columbia's brainy undergraduates who hailed from around the country and the world, but riding the subway to and from my classes, cramming for the good grades that would get me into medical school.

Medical school admission was like the Irish sweepstakes, a cutthroat rat race that saw a lot of the best and the brightest going to places like Guadalajara in Mexico, or Grenada in the Caribbean, or Grenoble in France, all schools of last resort when everywhere in America sent you a thin letter of rejection.

I ended up at Downstate Medical School in Brooklyn, part of the New York State University system. Downstate was one of the largest medical schools in the country, and one of the least glamorous, another subway school filled with the grandchildren of immigrants. But these kids were often brilliant, and Downstate was renowned for the quality of doctors it produced. I could have gone to Syracuse University, but I still didn't want to leave my mother, who was getting perceptibly weaker every year. I did take a room in the dorm, however, because of the intense nature of the program and the long subway ride from the Bronx to Brooklyn. I made the hour and a half (each way) trip home every weekend. There were times when I felt I shouldn't be getting my degrees from Columbia or Downstate but rather from the IRT (Interborough Rapid Transit), the IND (Independent Line), and the BMT (Brooklyn Manhattan Transit), the rapid transit lines (now phased out as distinct entities) that took me to school and back. I was underground for so much of my education that I felt like a subway vampire. Dostoyevsky's *Notes from the Underground* could have been the title of my collegiate autobiography.

Downstate wasn't much more cheerful than a subway station. There was no campus, no lawn, no trees, just buildings attached to the huge and charmless Kings County Hospital, which could have been in Communist Russia were it not for its high quality equipment and laboratories. This was no-frills education, but, to be fair, the uptown colossus that was Columbia Medical School wasn't that much better, except for its views over the Hudson. But charm wasn't the point, medicine was. Downstate had a truly distinguished faculty: world-class pioneers in heart transplants and kidney dialysis, a group of Nobel Prize winners, men to be inspired by, men to emulate. Medical school wasn't something to be enjoyed, but rather an ordeal to survive. That was the point, to toughen you up so you could endure anything. Medicine wasn't for sissies, I quickly learned.

There were two hundred students in my entering medical school class. We were either jammed into sloping amphitheatre-like auditoriums, being lectured to on subjects like physiology, biology, and pharmacology, or else herded into labs to work on cadavers. I called my first one "Gus" and found him to be a better friend to me than most of my intensely focused classmates. I frequently thought of the famous Rembrandt painting, *The Anatomy Lesson*, and how intimate, and personal it made medicine seem. Downstate was more like a factory, cold and impersonal with a distinct lack of human touch. Oddly enough, however, I liked the detachment of it all. I was a good student, and, like all good students, I was adept at memorizing things, which is what the first two years of medical school are all about. The final two were clinical, in that we were finally taken into the hospital and unleashed on real living humans. Until then, med school was an orgy of memory and anything but Proustian. Still, I was good at it, and being adept made me feel good.

I also fell in love. You really needed love in such a frigid environment, but I hardly expected to find it there. Until med school, I had enjoyed practically zero social life. Between commuting and studying, there wasn't much time to meet and court women. One summer at Columbia, my father got me a job through his Teamster contacts working on a delivery truck in the garment district. My overprotective mother, whose idea of a risky summer job was my being a camp counselor, was horrified, but to me it seemed masculine, tough, and cool, like Brando in *On the Waterfront*, and I just did it. I met some floor models and secretaries that summer, so I wasn't completely hopeless. Generally, though, the notions of lothario and pre-med were pretty mutually exclusive.

I met Elaine in the dorms, which were actually tiny apartments, rendering the need for gender segregation unnecessary. We didn't have to share bathrooms. She was an entering student when I was in my second year. Bobby Darin (an unlikely Bronx Science alum) had a song called "Queen of the Hop," and that's what Elaine was in her medical class. There were only twenty or so women out of the two hundred, and to say Elaine was by far the class beauty wasn't to damn her with faint praise. She would have been pretty anywhere. She was from Connecticut and had that tall, blonde, country club Greenwich look. But her looks were deceiving. Elaine was actually from the industrial town of New Britain, the daughter of Polish immigrants. He father worked in a tool factory. She had gone to Wellesley on a scholarship. She was an accomplished violinist. She was a pure shiksa, as opposite from the world I had grown up in as a woman could be. So, of course, we fell for each other.

The hitch was that I couldn't take her home to meet my parents. They always assumed I would marry a nice Jewish girl. I had gone to Connecticut to meet her parents, who were incredibly nice, but I kept making excuses, not wanting to blow my first full-blown romance over cultural issues.

In our rare free time, Elaine and I listened to classical music together, went for long walks on the promenade in Brooklyn Heights overlooking the spires of lower Manhattan, and played squash together. For medical school, I was something of a jock, having become a habitué of Downstate's one athletic facility: a squash court converted from a storage room. Squash was an essential stress-reliever, as was Elaine. She knew she was something of a babe and, self-esteem basher that I was, I never quite understood why she chose me. To commemorate our many dissections, I once gave her a pillow-sized stuffed toad, which she loved.

Our classmates used to call Elaine "princess" because she was so blonde and regal. She called me "toad," which was intended as endearing, not insulting, albeit not the stuff of self-esteem. The idea was that if she kissed me, she would turn this toad into a prince. Because she was the "Polish princess," my classmates, who openly and good-naturedly envied my being with Elaine, began calling me the "Polish prince," in reference to pop star Bobby Vinton, whose great hit was "Blue Velvet." I guess you had to be there, but it really was true love, med school-style.

By our third year, Elaine and I moved into a small apartment in Flatbush together. I still hadn't told my parents about my relationship, but I had stopped going back to the Bronx every weekend. My excuse was that I was in the clinical phase of med school, which was an around-the-clock forced march. It was hard to balance parents, a girlfriend, and this boot camp education, but somehow I managed. The idea was to suffer, become strong, and become a better doctor. I'm not so sure this was the case, but I did learn to survive on no sleep.

The third year was a series of rotations in the hospital: obstetrics, general surgery, psychiatry, internal medicine. I had no idea, at that point, what kind of doctor I wanted to be. Each field seemed worse than the next. But I was learning on the job, and I supposed the idea was to achieve grace under pressure. To me, med school seemed liked a fraternity hazing process that lasted not just for "hell week" but for four grueling years. My fellow students and I were like pledges, heads forced into toilets, only allowed to breathe when we were an inch from death. The attitude of most professors who chose to teach, rather than practice as real doctors, was that if they could survive the torture, so could you. Accordingly, they did their best to intimidate, humiliate, and destroy the spirit of any fledgling student who struggled to keep his head out of the toilet bowl.

One of my most painful memories occurred during the beginning of my OB-GYN rotation, or clinical clerkship, as it was called. On the first day of the program, three of my classmates and I arrived at the fourth floor maternity ward of Kings Hospital at 6:30 p.m., the normal starting time for most departments. Not there, alas. The supervising doctor, a snarling martinet named Eichenwald, was livid. His starting time was 6 p.m., and we had kept this great man waiting for a half hour. What were you doing for the last half hour, he demanded of us. When we told him we were eating dinner, he exploded with rage. "Eating? You were eating?" Eichenwald barked, as if it were a crime against nature. We were to be punished for this sin by being ordered to do hematocrits, or blood counts, on all the expecting mothers on the ward, about a hundred women ready to give birth, most of them screaming loudly. Most of the screamers were West Indians, Jamaicans, Trinidadians, and Anguillans, but their emanations were a cultural phenomenon of joy not pain. The ward, however, was far from joyous. It was totally Dickensian, reminding me of the Masterpiece Theatre series *Bramwell*. That 1890s London charity clinic seemed far superior to this one.

Dr. Eichenwald picked hematocrits because it was the meanest thing he could think of assigning to students who had never done one before, an intricate, time-consuming procedure where anything could, and usually did, go wrong. Taking small pins, we proceeded to draw blood from the fingers of the women, which gave them something else to scream about. None of us had any training in this: these women were our guinea pigs. Once we pricked the fingers and were able to massage a bead of blood out, our next task would be to suck that blood into a fragile, ultra-thin glass pipette about two inches tall. The other end of the pipette would be planted in clay to close it before putting it into a centrifuge. Of course, many of the pipettes broke, or the tags flew off, or the blood flew out. So more fingers had to be pricked, and there were a lot more screams.

It was bedlam; I wasn't sure who was having a more difficult time, the poor mothers-to-be or the poor doctors-to-be. However, by 8 a.m. the following morning, we always got the job done, messy and crazy as it was. Aside from pricking those endless fingers, we also had lots of scut work to do—taking urine samples, cleaning bedpans, taking patients for X-rays. Dr. Eichenwald's eyes gleamed with sadistic pleasure at our mounting frustration and exhaustion. The doctor, himself a resident only two years ahead of us, had probably experienced the same mistreatment by his superiors, and therefore felt it was his rightful turn to wreak his own vengeance on us. Such harassment would continue throughout my years as a medical student, intern, and resident. It was the proverbial rite of passage.

In addition to the fraternity hazing analogy, I also thought of the Algonquin Indians. A young boy would have to endure the initiation rites of manhood by passing through a gauntlet of adult braves brandishing clubs. As the boy crossed each adult, he would be battered. If he survived to the end of the line, he would become a brave and inherit the strength of his warrior ancestors. As a medical student, I was forced to take orders from my superiors, superiors who had endured abuse from their superiors, and on and on.

This ritualistic system of medical torture bred not only resentment but a sense of entitlement. Many physicians believe that because they have paid such onerous dues, the world owes them reparations in the form of an extremely good living. Sometimes, certainly before the advent of managed care, it seemed incongruous to regular people that a doctor should want to be paid so much for his services. The idea was that doctors should be like clergymen, practicing a noble calling for purely altruistic reasons. When I entered medical school, I saw doctors as our lay priests. The idea of their sporting tans and driving Porsches never occurred to me. But once I saw the suffering involved in the training process, I began to understand how this most humane of professions could lose its humanity.

I had to accept that this was medicine, for better or for worse; it was a good introduction to the crazed and imperfect system I would be entering. Soon I would be delivering these women's babies as well, which was quite a thrill, but not something I saw doing on a lifelong basis. I did like wearing the white doctor's coat, draping the stethoscope around my neck, carrying the little black bag. I thought I was Ben Casey or Dr. Kildare, and I felt important, a life-giver, a lifesaver.

I had never been so wiped out. Amazingly, I had the stamina to keep going. These were battlefield conditions, and I was ready to go to war. There were moments of praise, but for the most part, those shining moments were bracketed by humiliation, browbeating, and abusive, drill sergeant treatment by the more senior staff. None of it made me a better doctor, in my opinion.

Years later, New York State passed what was known as the Libby Zion Law, after the noted columnist's daughter died at a well-funded hospital on New York's glamorous Upper East Side due to the negligence of sleep-deprived residents. The law limited the number of hours a doctor could work. Fortunately, during my training, nothing tragic happened; still, I felt my training was at the expense of my many charity patients, who I hope still benefited from the trust they put in me, inadvertently or not. I was always fully aware of the enormous responsibility of someone's well-being, of life itself, and extended myself accordingly, often far beyond my body's capacity.

Fourth year of med school was more elective than third. I decided I liked psychiatry best of all the rotations my third year, especially after interviewing some seriously deranged characters at the Kings County Mental Institution. At least they had a bit of life in them, which was more than I could say for some of my professors. I had never seen so little emotion anywhere, and I was overwhelmed by the coldness of my learning experience. The one professor who truly touched me was my anatomy teacher; like my mother, he suffered from Parkinson's. His slight tremor made him seem vulnerable and human, though he never mentioned the illness and I wouldn't have dared mention it. Medical school was not a bonding process, to say the least.

Year after year, in medical schools across the country, and not just in cold, hard, fast New York, first-year classes enter, filled with a sense of privilege and excitement about becoming doctors. Four years later, the thrill is gone. All the enthusiasm has been beaten out of you. Excitement has given way to cynicism and numbness. By graduation, students have learned what they came for but forgotten why they came. By the end of school, I had lost the meaning of what I was doing, even though I was great at doing it. Proust wrote, "The voyage of discovery lies not in seeking new vistas, but in having new eyes." After medical school, mine were glazed over.

Throughout all my rotations, I was unclear as to where my career would go. As for Elaine, she stayed focused on her goal of becoming a surgeon. She had great hands—hands that made sweet music on the violin, hands that made delicate needlepoint, hands that would save lives someday. I loved those hands, and later on, once she had gotten her degree, when Elaine was addressed as "Mrs." Reiter, in the regal, formal English manner by the Chief of Surgery, I burst with pride, not only that she had taken my name, but also about the brilliant future she had ahead of her, of us.

Despite the public perception of med students as millionaires in training, we never, ever talked about how much money we would make. We were all living on next to nothing, and the idea of solvency, much less wealth, seemed light years away. Still, we all knew, as the public did, that doctors were often rich, which they were indeed, in those halcyon days before the rise of managed care and HMOs and red tape that strangled the profession. We lived in extreme pain but could take comfort in the distant prospect that, once we figured out what to do with our lives as doctors, we could count on financial security, if nothing else. But it still didn't seem real at the time, so we just soldiered on.

Later in my fourth year, I had an epiphany: I, too, wanted to become a surgeon. I decided I didn't want to sit on a couch and listen to other people's laments. No, I, who had been fairly passive all my life, decided I wanted, needed, to become a man of action. This didn't come from watching some Steve McQueen movie. This came from watching the real thing. Surgeons, I had observed in my rotation, were the most decisive of doctors. In modern parlance, they kicked ass. Even when they were short, frail, and directly off the boat from the old country, they seemed, by the very boldness of their actions, tall, muscular, big skyish, all-American heroes. They were real men in the best sense of the concept. Psychiatry was what I was. Surgery, just the opposite, was what most people would assume I never could be. So I went for it. I think I wanted to change my destiny.

To that end, I married Elaine at the office of a Justice of the Peace toward the end of the term. We went to Aruba for our honeymoon over spring break. I still didn't tell my parents, which deeply hurt Elaine, but not as much as I feared it would hurt my mother. I was trying to balance equities. Elaine could take the pain better than my mother could. Even when Elaine threw a big party for my graduation at Gage and Tollner, a wonderful century-old seafood restaurant in Brooklyn with gas lamps and venerable black waiters, totally out of the Gilded Age, I still couldn't break the news to my folks. We pretended to be school chums.

My brother, Ira, showed up at the party. He had just gotten married himself, to Suzyn, a stunning Jewish carpet-store heiress from Scarsdale, who had set him up in the wine business, at which he was making a fortune. My parents were totally delighted with him. So much for studying night and day, and riding the subway to the end of our youth. Oh, well. I couldn't be jealous. I had a great wife and a great future as a surgeon. Who could ask for anything more, other than maybe being able to tell my family about it? I had done the greatest thing an old world son could do: become a doctor. And I had done the worst, too: marry a shiksa.

My next step on my road to becoming a surgeon was a one-year internship, which was another boot camp, totally hands-on. Again, I had no option but to stay in New York. Elaine had one more year at Downstate, and my mother continued to need me. So I went back to the Bronx, to the extremely prestigious Albert Einstein Medical Center. I was lucky—honored—to have been accepted as one of thirty interns from all over the world. Ironically, this was where my mother came for her Parkinson's follow-ups. We were now both in the same place. I hoped that by being on the inside, I could find some brilliant doctor who could find a miracle cure for her. But I wasn't banking on it. The doctor/professors of Downstate showed me how distances were made to be kept. Unlike Downstate, which was prewar industrial, Einstein was gleamingly modern, if not futuristic. Elaine and I found an apartment nearby, from which she would make the endless subterranean slog every day to Brooklyn. I can never thank her enough for having made such a big sacrifice for me, but she knew that an internship was even more grueling than med school, so she took the bullet.

As nice as Einstein itself was, Jacoby and Lincoln, the city hospitals with which it was affiliated, and where I would spend my days and nights, were the medical equivalent of *Blackboard Jungle*. If emergencies were the surgical intern's trial by fire, these two hospitals provided the best test a young doctor could have, a festival of stab wounds, slashed throats, gouged out eyeballs, a true circus of horrors. Lincoln Hospital had actually been briefly taken over, in a siege, by the Young Lords, the most vicious of the Puerto Rican street gangs that were making the Bronx so dangerous that my parents had to move to an apartment across the Hudson in Fort Lee, New Jersey.

Jacoby Hospital was so primitive it seemed like a Civil War operating theater. There were huge open wards with twenty metal beds to a ward. There were green, faded tile walls, cracked linoleum floors, flimsy lace curtains, no privacy whatsoever. All that was needed to complete the primitive scene were a bunch of nuns in nurses' habits ministering to the poor and wounded. But I was the nun, and somehow, I really liked it. The program started in July, and the hospitals weren't air-conditioned. But the heat added to the sense of urgency, and urgency is what a surgeon thrives on. The philosophy of interning is: "See one, do one, teach one." The intern had to observe residents above him in action, then learn how to do it by being thrown into the fire, and then impart their new knowledge to the med students below him. It was a food chain, and it was eat or be eaten.

I delivered a lot of babies, and I sewed up a lot of wounds. I'll never forget cutting into a live human body for the first time. I must have read about the routine operation at least a hundred times before I took the plunge with every *Ben Casey* episode I had ever seen flashing before me. But once the knife went in, it felt like the most natural thing in the world. "This is where I belong!" I said to myself, exultantly. I had steady hands, and the sight of blood didn't disturb me. I was surgeon material. Bring on the patients!

And they did. I'd start every morning at 6 a.m., holding the skin retractors for the real surgeons during these long operations, watching, watching, watching, like a hawk with an elephant's memory. I didn't want to miss a trick, or to forget one. I would make rounds with the surgeon to his patients, and then take over for him. I'd change wound dressings, exchange IVs, place and replace catheters. By evening I would spend most of the hard day's night at the operating room, rising to emergencies as well as being on call for twenty to thirty post-op patients. This was where I learned to be a human version of an all-night diner, and I found I thrived on the deprivation of it all, in the name of health, the health of others. It was great getting outside myself, learning to give rather than receive. The old clichés, the Bible stuff, really worked.

The internship year went by in a flash. I was working so hard that I never noticed the calendar. Suddenly it was time to look for a residency, the final long step before going out on my own into practice. Surgical residencies are the hardest in medicine. They last five years. The best general surgery residency in New York, as far as I could determine, was at Mt. Sinai Hospital, on Fifth Avenue at 98th Street, just across from Central Park. Mt. Sinai was known to the legions of viewers of the film *Love Story* as the hospital where Ryan O'Neal got the grim news that Ali MacGraw was dying of cancer.

In general, the premier hospitals in Manhattan were Columbia Presbyterian, far up in Washington Heights, and New York Hospital-Cornell Medical Center, in the far east 60s, but Mt. Sinai was the king for general surgery. I had done very well at Einstein, and, although I had made no real friends or mentors, I did garner a lot of respect, and great recommendations got me into the coveted residency. Meanwhile, Elaine was able to secure an internship at Flower Fifth Avenue-New York Medical College Hospital. Flower Fifth, as it was known, had been a movie star as well, playing itself in *The Hospital*, starring George C. Scott, a broadside against the medical profession written by Paddy Chayefsky, who did a similar broadside against television years later in *Network*. Elaine and I kept our apartment in the Bronx near Einstein and drove into Manhattan every morning in a hot Buick Riviera my father had gotten for next to nothing from one of his gangster friends. Once Elaine graduated, I broke the news of my marriage to my folks, and it wasn't as bad as I had expected. The Riviera was his wedding gift to us, and as my very first car, my first symbol of extravagance, and with my MD plates, I thought I was pretty hot stuff. So did a policeman who pulled me over for running a stop sign and refused to accord me doctor's immunity. "I guess your wife has the Cadillac today," he said to me, writing out a hefty fine. I wanted to say to him, "When you're shot in the neck, you're going to need me," but I held my tongue.

I spent the first two months of my residency with a famed breast cancer surgeon known among his peers as "The Hangman." He was expressionless and heartless. This was before implants. The doctor had no bedside manner whatsoever. He never prepared his patients for what might happen. He was there to save their lives, not to deal with their self-image. He'd put these poor patients under anesthesia in those pre-mammogram days to do the biopsy, and half of them would wake up missing one or both breasts. Hey, I got your cancer, is how he would look at it. I wasn't about to question him. While less of a death march than the internship, residency was pretty much an Army kind of experience. The hangman was the general, and I was the grunt private, and that's the way it was. Sensitivity was for girls and hippies, not surgeons.

Then Elaine had her own cancer scare. A PAP smear indicated dysplasia of the cervix. She needed to get a biopsy. I wanted to be by my wife's side during what I was sure would be a traumatic ordeal, but The Hangman refused to let me off to be with her. "It's nothing," he said without knowing a thing. "You have your responsibilities here." He was as mean and without feeling as Dr. Eichenwald on the charity ward. Plus he was being mean about my wife. I felt angry, ashamed, and guilty about even thinking about not going with Elaine. But Elaine wouldn't let me. She was a good soldier, too, and she knew the drill. She insisted on going alone. Her courage, and her insistence on "taking it like a man," made me love her all the more. She was so proud to be a doctor, and to be married to one, that she insisted we do whatever the system, awful as it was, required of us.

It turned out The Hangman was right about its being nothing. The biopsy was negative. The Hangman was always right, as far as he was concerned. That's why he was a star. But I still hated him and vowed I would never treat my patients the way he did. When I was covering his patients, I wanted to give them hope, but nothing is crueler than false hope. Furthermore, even if, in my very inexperienced opinion, the lump in question was benign, I dared not voice that opinion on the off chance it was malignant. I was too young, too green to shoot from the hip. All I could do was to assure them they were in the hands of a fine doctor who could rise to whatever the occasion was. But so often when they awoke breastless, the aftermath was devastating. The main thing I learned from my first rotation was that I didn't want to be a breast surgeon.

On another early rotation, in heart surgery, at the Mt. Sinai affiliated Bronx Veterans Hospital, I was amazed at the low level of care the patients who had been heroes in World War II or the Korean War and were now being treated like low priority charity cases. "Hey, it's the Veterans hospital," said the fat, slovenly chief of surgery there. That same chief, however, who would skimp on patient surgery, knew how to exploit government grants for furnishings and office equipment. If a budget of $1 million came down from Washington, he would spend it on a warehouse of pencils and memo pads or cigars and cigarettes and artery-clogging candy bars for his cardiology staff rather than send the excess back. There was tremendous waste and misallocation, stuff right out of Joseph Heller's *Catch-22*. Luckily, these rotations didn't last forever, or my outrage might have made me ill.

I wasn't what I would call a whistle-blower, but as a doctor, taxpayer, and hospital worker, I felt honor-bound to at least speak my mind about the abuses of the system I witnessed. So I screwed up my courage and went to the chief of the VA Hospital to speak my piece. Instead of showing any interest in what I told him, he gave me a lecture on the way the system worked and strongly suggested I get used to it or go find another system to work in. I was so frustrated that I actually called the Veterans Administration in Washington DC. I ended up venting my spleen at some secretary, who told me to save my breath and put it in a letter, which I did. I never got a reply.

I was learning what kind of surgeon I didn't want to be, but I still hadn't found my true calling. Just as in med school, there was little sense of community among the residents at the hospital. It wasn't exactly every man for himself, but in medicine, almost every doctor is on his own, so unless you were jockeying to get on a professorial track at Harvard or some other important research center, you were really there to take the knowledge and run. We were under so much stress, with so many patients and so little time, that we didn't have the strength, much less the hours, to think about our ambitions. It really was like being at war; the best we could hope to do was display grace under pressure.

I did make one good friend, a lanky, farmboyish fellow named Dennis Gans from Ames, Iowa. I used to joke that Dennis was one of the three Jews in the Midwest before I discovered that there was life west of the Hudson, which I had still never ventured beyond in my subwaycentric existence. Dennis's father had had a successful clothing store in their small town. His brother had become an ear, nose, and throat surgeon, and Dennis was following in his footsteps. Somehow Dennis's enthusiasm for ENT proved to be catching, and I got excited at the notion of restoring people's hearing. My Aunt Shirley, my mother's sister, whom I liked very much, was partially deaf, and I had watched her suffering for years. The idea of being able to do something about it, to break new medical ground perhaps, was intriguing to me.

I thus went to the chief of otolaryngology at Mt. Sinai to see if I could get into his specialized residency program, which was where Dennis Gans was. Alas, he told me he was completely filled up. The next opening would not be before two years. I could continue in my five-year general surgery residency, but, since I now knew what I wanted to specialize in, that would be a waste of time. So I began to look for other programs, no easy task since most young doctors had planned their lives far better than I. The few spots available were already taken. Elaine, whose grueling internship at Flower Fifth and the patronizingly sexist treatment she was getting there ("How many babies do you plan to have?" colleagues asked. "How long do you plan to stay a doctor?") were making her question her career in medicine, had the bright idea of my finding a program in Paris or London, where she could chuck the whole medicine bit, at least for a while, and join a symphony. That seemed too radical to me; besides, cautious Jewish husband that I was, I didn't want Elaine to give up the brilliant career ahead of her. But then Dennis Gans offered up an opportunity that would keep us both on American soil.

Dennis had gone to medical school at the University of Iowa. One of the faculty giants there, Leslie Bernstein, a South African ENT-plastic surgeon whom Dennis had gotten to know, had just gone out to a new chair at the University of California at Davis. One of his residents had just come down with tuberculosis and had to drop out. Perhaps I could take his place. I thus flew out to San Francisco in April, rented a car at the airport, and drove the two hours to Davis, outside the capital of Sacramento. Although I had never been to California, it was so etched in the public consciousness as America's Promised Land that I felt I knew it well. The Haight-Ashbury Summer of Love had just occurred a few years before. The Mamas and the Papas sang "California Dreamin'." And the Beach Boys never stopped their endless odes to the endless summer of the Golden State.

While the April I left in New York was one of melting snow and slush, sleet, and cold rain, California was eternal spring. Davis, in California's agriculturally bountiful Central Valley, was a farmers' paradise: verdant, balmy, and fragrant, something I had never known. I was entranced with the open spaces, the newness, the cleanliness of it all. Davis was a showcase campus of the University of California, and Leslie Bernstein was a showcase professor. Small and physically unprepossessing, Leslie was instantly a giant in my eyes. He was the most self-confident person I had ever met, and he used his London-polished South African accent to great effect. He might have looked like Danny DeVito, but the minute he opened his mouth, he became Lord Mountbatten. We spent about five hours together, with Leslie showing me the campus and grilling me about what I knew and what I could do and how obsessively I could work. He must have been pleased, because by the end of the day, he offered me the "tubercular" opening. He wanted me there on July 1, just months away. I hesitated, thinking about New York, thinking about my mother, and then I realized that hesitation wasn't in Leslie's lexicon. So I accepted the offer on the spot.

I spent the long trip home rationalizing what I had done. I spent the night in San Francisco wandering up and down the foggy hills, riding the cable cars, eating chop suey alone in a decrepit but delicious dive in Chinatown. What was there not to like? Only my mother, my poor mother, I despaired. But then I tried to be rational. She had my father, my brother, her seven brothers and sisters, to whom she was close, all in New York. It wasn't as if I were abandoning her to the wolves. She would be fine. I wasn't betraying her by leaving. Besides, I was going to work with Leslie Bernstein, the god of facial plastic surgery. I wasn't sure my mother ever took my becoming a surgeon seriously. She was big on Jews "knowing their places," and one of those places was not being a surgeon, which was strictly for WASPs, in her Bronx worldview. I would have loved for her to meet Leslie, to rebut all her presumptions. I was doing this for her, as much as for me, to prove to her the kind of man her little boy could be.

Back in slushy New York, I tried to inflame Elaine with the lure of the Golden West. "Sacramento?" was all she could ask. It wasn't a big musical town, nor was it big on culture in general. But I kept stressing how close San Francisco was. "The Metropolitan Opera's just across the park, and how many times have we gone?" she asked, resting her case. At the same time, I was contacted by another world-famous ENT surgeon: Dr. Fitzhugh of the University of Virginia, who wanted me to know about an opening to be his resident. Obviously, Virginia was a lot closer to home than California, and Elaine would have preferred it. But I had given Leslie my word, and that was that. In any event, I was beyond flattered that two dominant figures in my future field had given me their vote of confidence. That recognition did not soften the news when I broke it to my mother. She thought she was losing me forever, and I had to work overtime to assure her that I'd be back.

When Elaine and I arrived in Sacramento at the end of June, the world looked totally different than it did back in April. The eternal spring had become an infernal summer, with temperatures over 110 degrees. All the greenery had turned desert brown, parched and dried out. It wasn't the California of our dreams. Luckily we had spent the week before in

San Francisco, so we knew the dream wasn't a total fantasy. We had left the Buick Riviera back in New York and now bought a rickety used Plymouth Scamp to get around in. We also bought, for twenty thousand dollars, a little Craftsman bungalow near the Davis campus. There were cows in the field across the road, too enervated by the heat to move, but I kept telling Elaine it was far more nature than we'd ever see in New York. She just turned on the air conditioner and retreated into her classical music. She was able to get a job at the Kaiser hospital in family planning. She was earning about twenty thousand dollars a year. I was getting a stipend of ten, which would have to see me through each of the next four years of my ENT-facial plastic surgery surgical residency. In addition to his requiring a two years' general surgery residency, Leslie's own program was a year longer than everyone else's, for a total of six years of residency, but that was part of the honor. Heaven, and any high living, would obviously have to wait.

I hit the ground running. Leslie, field commander martinet that he was, insisted on superhuman performance and endurance. He constantly demanded the impossible, like an overnight treatise on all the most recent developments in thyroid cancer in time for the next morning's crack-of-dawn surgery. The order came at 9 p.m.; he wanted my paper at 6 a.m. the following morning, when we began our rounds. At first I protested. How could I do a major research project in nine hours, allowing only a few hours for sleep. "Sleep!" he said with a dismissive laugh, just as dismissive as Dr. Eichenwald had been about food. Lives depended on me, he told me, and I stretched my limits accordingly. I was obsessive compulsive to begin with, so the idea of letting my mentor down was anathema to me. I worked all night. He loved the paper.

Even though I thought I'd go into ENT to become a hearing surgeon, it turned out that Leslie's great forte was maxillo-facial surgery, or restoring destroyed faces, and that eventually became my sphere of interest as well. Originally trained as a dentist in Durban, Leslie had gone on to London and become a star there, and was lured to America by the huge research grants lavished upon him. America had money for medicine that was unmatched anywhere else in the world. Still, there was a part of Leslie that was wistful, if not ashamed, about selling out to come and live in the sticks, first the cornfields of Iowa and now these cow pastures in Davis. He had fine art in his office, where, with Handel in the background, he would pour his guests vintage French wines and pretend he was still on Harley Street. However homesick he may have been for old world civilization, he never once complained about where he was. That would have been a display of weakness, and a great surgeon never whined.

In the beginning I had reason to whine but, following Leslie's example, I never did. On my first day in the ER, I had two patients with displaced zygomas, or cheekbones. They were an older couple who had been assaulted when someone tried to steal the wife's purse. The husband and wife had identical fractures. The attending doctor examined them with me, took me out of the ER, told me what to do, and then left for dinner. I thus had these two people's faces in my hands, hands that had never fixed a facial fracture without supervision before. Fortunately, I was a quick study. Using an open textbook, I was able to reduce both their fractures successfully.

Only afterward, after the adrenalin had worn off, did I get angry. How dare an attending doctor leave a complete novice alone to fix these poor, unsuspecting people's faces. If a fracture is not restored properly the first time, there's rarely a second chance. It's a one shot, best shot deal. And a facial fracture has to be fixed correctly within a certain time frame. If not, the bones will mend, and they will have to be rebroken and grafts taken from the hip and…in short, it's a catastrophe. I was good, to be sure, but still. He shouldn't have done that. But there was no time to contemplate the alternatives. It was do or die, quite literally.

Another even more extreme example comes to mind in relation to the "see one, do one, teach one" mentality that permeated medical training. I had been called in by the resident fellow one evening to attend to the victim of a shotgun blast. The poor patient looked like a bloody Andy Gump, his entire jaw fragmented and missing, with a loss of the surrounding skin and the floor of his mouth. All that was left was a trembling portion of tongue. When I called the attending doctor, the same one who had left me alone with those two facial fractures, to ask his supervision over me and the resident who was there with me, he said he was having dinner. "I think you can handle it," he said. "Call me if you have any problems." And he hung up.

Once again there was no time for anger or outrage. Twelve hours later, my colleague and I had managed to sew this unfortunate man's face back together. We stayed up all night reconstructing his mouth and tongue, controlling the bleeding and removing bits of shattered jawbone. It was like putting the pieces of a jigsaw puzzle together, except many of those pieces were lying on a dark California highway. In all those hours of surgery, I felt like part of *The Cabinet of Doctor Caligari*, but I was breaking new ground, and Leslie loved that. After hours of surgery, the next step was to create enough tissue by bringing up flaps from his neck and chest so as to be able to put the new jawbone in place. It took months for this initial surgery to heal. This surgery was always accompanied by apprehension and pain for the patient, although we always tried to be as reassuring as possible. After the skin and muscle grafting healed, I put the new jawbone in.

I completely won Leslie's respect when I proposed putting in a total jaw transplant, using the jawbone of a cadaver. Obviously there were no live donors who could spare their jawbones the way there might be for a kidney or bone marrow transplant. I eventually used a freshly obtained freeze-dried mandible, or jawbone, of a cadaver in the later reconstruction of the lower third of this victim's face.

This, I believe, was the first time such a transplant had been done, and while it worked fine for aesthetic purposes, functionally, the man would never be able to chew food again. I was sad about that, but my work did lead the way to new, innovative treatments for people with cancer of the mandible and other facial bones.

I would have done a paper on it, but I was working too hard to write up anything. One night alone I had to operate on four different jaw fractures. The Sacramento Delta was the world capital of jaw fractures, a violent Wild West place where Mexican migrant workers used their fists to the same lethal effect that the Puerto Ricans in the Bronx used their switchblades and ice picks. The Mexicans also used hammers, clubs, and whatever farm implements they could lay their hands on. Unlike in the Bronx, where drugs were always concomitant to the violence, in the Delta, old-fashioned alcohol, mescal or tequila, was the inebriant of choice. Most of the domestic white violence involved shotguns, and I recreated many a jaw that had been blown away.

The Night of Four was one of the rare times I simply fell apart. I was totally fatigued to begin with, and as the bodies rolled in, I was overwhelmed: by the volume of work, by the terrible stench of blood and alcohol (the victims were all inebriated), by the twelve hours ahead of me looking into mouths, tongues, teeth, saliva, blood. The patients were lined up, sitting in dental chairs. They needed me desperately. Yet I didn't think I could summon up the energy to set another fracture. Jaw fractures are repaired with what is known as a "closed reduction," in which the teeth are wired with archbars, which are then wired together, locking the jaw shut. After the jaw is wired like this, the patient survives by drinking fluids, sucking them between his teeth for a six-week period. It seems like torture, but that's what it takes to live.

I went into an empty lounge to catch my breath, but instead I lost it. I broke down in tears, which is the last thing a doctor is expected to do. I cried alone for a few minutes. Was I weak? Unmanly? Self-indulgent? Would Hippocrates have cried? Would Ben Casey? I didn't care. I needed it. A dam had broken, and I just went with the feelings, the myriad emotions that had been suppressed during these endless years of macho medical boot camp. And then the crying stopped. I dried my eyes, splashed cold water on my face, downed a cup of black coffee, and returned to work to put those people back together.

Leslie's only other first-year resident was his nephew Edward. They only spoke to each other in Afrikaans, and I thought there was no way I would ever become Leslie's Number One. I got my break when it was discovered that Edward had a foreign licensing problem and wasn't allowed to take emergency calls. Of necessity, I became Leslie's right hand. Maybe being the only other Jew in the program endeared me to him, but Leslie never said a Yiddish phrase to me. That was beneath his Anglo-ness, yet I did sense a bond somehow beneath his pomp and circumstance.

Leslie trusted me enough to send me to Los Angeles as his emissary to research a new temporal bone laboratory that he had gotten a huge grant to build. I flew down to Los Angeles to visit the House Institute, connected to St. Vincent's Hospital, which, at the time, was the premier ear surgery center in the nation. Howard House, the founder, was a father of modern ear surgery. This was my first visit to fabled Los Angeles. What I was expecting was Beverly Hills; what I got was Tijuana. St. Vincent's was located near downtown in what seemed to be a Mexican barrio. I had to dodge a gauntlet of panhandlers just to get into the place. Deafening mariachi music filled the air, as did the smell of stale taco grease. There was awful smog and awful traffic. It was like the South Bronx with palm trees. I concentrated on the microscopes and other equipment we would be buying to set up the Davis lab.

I spent an anxious night at a dingy place actually called the Notel Motel listening to police sirens. The next day I took a cab straight back to the airport. I didn't have the time to do a tour of the homes of the stars, or go see Grauman's Chinese Theater. Surgeons like me had no time for such frivolities. My first impression of the city was so inauspicious that I couldn't imagine ever living there.

I had won Leslie's respect, and I respected him greatly, but Elaine hated him. Once, when we were out on a tennis court trying to have a life, my pager went off for the tenth time and Elaine broke down in tears. She hated her job at Kaiser, seeing a patient every six minutes. Her original dreams of surgery had fallen by the wayside of exigency, her great hands notwithstanding. Elaine especially hated never seeing me. She thought I loved Leslie more than I loved her. But no one loved Leslie; they feared him. He had ruined many a resident's life by firing them abruptly midterm, giving them nowhere else to go.

And he was terribly cheap, despite his department's deep pockets. The first year I was there, I called my mother briefly every day from the department office. When he scrutinized the phone bills and found out I was making these long-distance calls, he got furious and ordered me to stop. I was wasting his money, and his time, he snarled. There were lives to save. My mother's didn't fall within his scope. Leslie tolerated nothing but perfection, and took all the credit for whatever you accomplished. He was also a Type A male chauvinist pig (the chief feminist epithet of the times) and treated women as appendages, including his charming wife, who always stood reverentially in his long shadow at department events. She, like everyone else, was there to reflect his glory. Once at a department soiree, he blustered to Elaine, "You're lucky I'm going to make Alvin a great surgeon."

"He is a great surgeon," she snapped, and turned on her heel. She didn't want his largesse, and she despised his chauvinism. Still, for me, he was a genius and a role model, for medicine, if not life. His endless encouragement made my career.

And so it went for the next four years, which were a lightning round of trauma, triumph, and the steepest learning curve in medicine I have ever experienced. One week alone I did sinus surgery, a tonsillectomy, a thyroidectomy, a rhinoplasty, an otoplasty, a blepharoplasty, three jaw replacements, and two grossly displaced cheekbone fractures. At that point I could truly say, "I have become a surgeon now."

But I still didn't necessarily get any respect. For example, when working with a patient with a severed trachea from a knife wound, I put in something called a Montgomery tube as a stent to keep the trachea open. I thought that I ingeniously put in two sutures connected to tiny "buttons" I implanted in the skin of the neck to prevent the stent from falling out and down into the lungs. Paul Donald, Leslie's second in command, a six-foot-six hawkish, bald Canadian from the prairies of

Manitoba, asked, "Who did this?" When I volunteered proudly that it was my handiwork, Paul attacked me. He said it would never work, the buttons would erode, the stent would fall out, all the worst things would happen. I had gotten it all wrong by putting the buttons outside the skin.

Instead of falling on my sword, however, I called Dr. Wayne Montgomery of Mass General, Harvard Medical School's teaching hospital, and asked the inventor of the stent bearing his name how he did it. Outside, he assured me. I never confronted Paul with the awful (for him) truth. However, when Leslie, who kept scrutinizing all the phone bills, asked every resident who had wasted department money by calling Boston, I had no choice but to admit the call, and no choice but to explain why. Paul was sitting right there, and turned red. But he never apologized. To him, as to Leslie, being a surgeon meant never having to say you're sorry.

To Paul Donald's credit, however, he did teach me one very valuable lesson about perseverance. Surgeries, especially with labor-intensive reconstruction, can take many, many hours. I was a hard worker to begin with, but I was being further molded in a crucible of fire, this time surgery fire. I recall starting a surgery involving cancer of the throat, jaw, tongue, and neck at 7 a.m. one morning. I was doing the surgery with the help of another surgical resident and the guidance of Paul Donald. Donald went home, as expected, later in the day and checked on our progress every few hours.

Believe it or not, we found ourselves, not unexpectedly, still at work at 7 a.m. the next morning. Fortunately these types of surgeries did not occur often. Our mentor and sometimes "tormenter" (for the good of the patient—always for the good of the patient) returned. Seeing me a little peaked, totally exhausted, but still standing, sewing, and cutting and about to finish this hopefully life-saving procedure. Donald gave me a quick lesson on the meaning of hope.

"You know, Alvin," he said in his Calgary Canadian accent, "this patient may have only a one in forty chance of surviving the cancer, but you do not know if you have that particular one in forty patient under your knife. Lesson: Do all you can despite the odds, no matter how hopeless a case may be. That patient has put his life in your hands." That lesson set a very high standard for me, and it would cause great heartache later in my life when I tried to hold other doctors to it.

I did my first facelift at Davis and discovered I had a true knack for it. I became fascinated with the structure of the face and read endless books on aesthetics, going back to the ancient Greeks. Eventually, I felt as if I had Superman-like X-ray vision of a person's skull, an ability to see through the skin to the bones, and to visualize how I could rewire nature's work to create the symmetry that was known as beauty. I learned about the harmony of the relationships between upper and lower jaws, the angles between the nose and lips, the distances between eyes. Medicine thus became art, and Leslie, who was a master of aesthetics, was the perfect mentor. He was also an artist: he insisted that I take drawing classes. So every Thursday night I became, not an overwhelmed young surgeon, but a bohemian artist sketching models and dreaming of Paris in the '20s, where I would hang out with Picasso in Montmartre over a glass of absinthe. It was a fantasy respite from the blown-off faces and shattered jaws of the rest of every week. And those art classes taught me a lot.

It soon gave me great pleasure to be able to reconstruct a nose. It wasn't cutting off a nose to spite a face, but to make a face. I loved the way I could bring such joy into a patient's life. It may have seemed superficial to some people to acknowledge the importance of looks, but those were the facts of life. I may have come to Davis thinking my joy would be in making people hear better, but by the time I was ready to leave, that joy was in making them look better, and it did not diminish my self-esteem in the least. I discovered that plastic surgery had a long and noble tradition that I was proud to be joining.

Back in ancient India, for example, a widely accepted form of corporal punishment for thieves was amputation of the tip of the nose. An Indian surgeon named Sushata Samgita in 600 B.C. surgically reshaped these noses, making it possible for convicts to get a fresh start and not be stigmatized, as was literally as-clear-as the-nose-off-your-face case. Hindu surgeons became so skilled in reattaching these severed appendages that penal officials would throw the amputated noses into a fire to destroy them, so as to ensure the goal of disfigurement. Ironically, the skilled surgeons who were responsible for these underground criminal "nose jobs" were members of a lowly caste of potters, who seemed predestined to perform this task because of their sense of form and expression, as well as their capability to sculpt. It was a long way to the pinnacle of Beverly Hills or Rio or Paris society, where plastic surgeons had become Pygmalion-like gods.

At the end of the program, Leslie and I decided I should go into academia. I was already a full-time member of the Davis faculty, enjoying all the honors that title bestowed, including a parking space in the faculty lot. Academics made sense for me. I read voraciously about every obscure aspect of my specialty, and I loved sharing my knowledge with other residents, as well as interns and medical students. When I expressed an interest in staying in teaching, Leslie couldn't have been more thrilled. It was an ego boost to his already huge ego to have a disciple in academe spreading his word. Accordingly, he arranged professor track teaching positions in maxilo-facial reconstructive surgery at Columbia and Harvard medical schools. I was flattered beyond belief, and for the first time in our four years at Davis, Elaine was overjoyed, chiefly at the prospect of returning to civilization. Leslie liked the idea of placing one of his acolytes in a position of power in the Ivy League, and I was his man. It was pretty heady, the idea of being Professor Reiter.

But a funny thing happened on my way to Harvard: Beverly Hills came calling. Actually the call came from Birmingham, Alabama, where my friend Dennis Gans, who had sent me to Davis to begin with, had set up an ENT practice and was loving it. He also loved the South. Dennis had a friend, Bill Manning, a distinguished ENT professor at Mt. Sinai, who had left New York to go into private practice in Beverly Hills. Manning, Gans told me, was from a rich family and wanted to enjoy his heritage before he got too old. He was tired of slogging through the New York winters and through the not-always-tropical groves of academe. Ganz suggested I go see him about joining his practice in Lotusland.

At that point, I had only been to LA once, and it didn't seem very Lotus-y to me. I knew Elaine regarded it, sight unseen, with the same contempt that Woody Allen, and many inveterate New Yorkers, held for it. To Elaine, it was the Wasteland, a cultural desert, an endless Disneyland of superficiality, stupid trends, and Manson cults. But then, I started thinking, not so much about the place, but about my life. All of a sudden, I was curious about private practice. At Harvard or Columbia, I would have had to be full-time faculty. I wouldn't be allowed to have any private patients. I would have huge prestige and zero money. At best I would have gotten a salary of $20,000 a year. That was twice my draw at Davis, but still, it was subsistence living. On a pro rata basis, plumbers made far more. I had been in school all my life, and had never seen the light of day, a normal, non-crisis, high-pressure, life-and-death day. As a professor I would have to go through what I had just gone through all over again, higher up the food chain perhaps, but still the same drill. I would have to take residents through the slashed throats and the tonsillectomies and the jaw fractures. Fatigue set in. Maybe man, medical man, couldn't live on prestige alone.

I spent a lot of time on the phone to Dennis Gans in Alabama, who sang the praises of private practice. I didn't have to go to Beverly Hills, he said. That was just one opening. What about Birmingham? They could use another smart Yankee. I thought about those other smart Yankees, Goodman, Chaney, and Schwerner, who had been murdered in adjacent Mississippi that "freedom summer" a few years before, and I begged off. Not that genteel Old South Birmingham was bad, but somehow it simply didn't have the magical allure of Beverly Hills. Not wanting to alarm Elaine, who was getting excited about the Harvard idea, I rang up Bill Manning in Beverly Hills just to feel out the situation. It was a false alarm, an illusory opportunity. "Don't bother," he told me. "I can't take the stuffy noses and sore throats. There's no challenge here. I'm getting rid of this practice and moving to Boston myself. See you at Harvard."

Somehow, Manning and I kept talking. I had this idea of private practice in my head now, and I wanted to play it out. So Manning referred me to the doctor he was selling his practice to, a drawly Texan named John Lipton, who had been his partner. "Don't listen to Bill,"

Lipton said to me. "He's a professor, not a doctor. Guy can't handle a good time. You'll love it here, best practice, best life, best living. Come on down, boy. We need you here."

And I did, just to take a look, much to Elaine's chagrin. She counted on my good taste to be appalled by what I would see. She just knew I would hate it, and the trip to Beverly Hills would ensure our hightailing it to Boston, its spiritual opposite. Of course, I loved it. Lipton was charming and laid back, but with an impressive resume. The practice he had taken over from Manning had been started by the recently retired Henry Rubin, throat doctor to the stars. Lipton wasn't a name-dropper, but he couldn't help but mention a dozen Oscar winners that he took care of. Star names were the great "signifier" of Los Angeles. If you treated stars, you were a star.

Lipton put me up at the brand new Century Plaza Hotel in brand new Century City, which had been built on part of the 20th Century Fox lot that had to be sold off when television began devouring the movies. Lipton had an office there in one of the skyscrapers. He had another office, which would become my office, in old Beverly Hills. After Sacramento and the cows, I was impressed by the urbanity of the place, combined with the luxury and comfort. There were skyscrapers, but they were surrounded by golf courses and palm trees. There were sophisticated restaurants, and even a great Jewish deli, Nate 'n Al's, where I saw Doris Day and Sid Caesar when Lipton took me there for a bagels and lox breakfast. It was all that New York had, minus the bad weather and the crime and the grafitti-covered subways, which I had endured enough of for three lifetimes. Even my parents had left the city for New Jersey.

Speaking of New York, my mother had been doing fine without me. I had gone back to see her on every one of my paltry two-week holidays, and all was as well as I could have hoped for. New Jersey wasn't Beverly Hills, but it was safe and the family was there. I was no longer consumed with guilt about not being within subway distance. The way Lipton made it sound, in the humane practice I would have, I would have more time to go back East to see her than I would if I were teaching in "we never close" Boston. And he would start me at a princely salary of $3,000 a month. It was an offer I couldn't refuse.

I'm not sure who was more livid, Elaine or Leslie Bernstein, who threatened, seriously, to fail me on my national ENT-facial plastic surgery medical boards, for which he was one of the chief examiners, and thus terminate my brilliant private career before it could begin. He wanted a man in the East, I think, to pave the way for his own triumphal arrival there. I was raining on the parade he was planning for himself. But I wouldn't let Leslie rain on *my* parade. Surgeons had to be decisive, and I played true to type. And eventually Elaine came around. I convinced her to give Beverly Hills a chance. She had become interested in singing, and Lipton got us a list of world-class vocal coaches with whom Elaine could study. Kaiser had offices in Los Angeles, and they would let her transfer. For once we would be a two-income family. "I went to medical school to marry a doctor," Elaine joked, and now that joke could become a reality. She was married to a real Beverly Hills doctor. We sold our bungalow, packed up the Scamp, and drove south to our brave new life.

Chapter Three

SCAMP

Dexter Farnham and I spent over an hour walking around the lush residential blocks between Beverly and Olympic boulevards, near the Surgery Center. We stayed away from Beverly Drive itself, with its trendy outdoor cafes, because to me that street had ears. The FBI visit had put me in a state of shock. I was instantly paranoid. I worried that my office, my house, my car had all been bugged. Aside from my cancer, I was used to a placid, highly controlled existence, my practice, my wife, my home and gardens. We had four cats. No children, no dogs, no turmoil. Everything was quiet, serene. In one fell swoop, the FBI had transformed that tranquility into a roaring, stomach-churning, sadistic amusement park ride.

"It's all politics," Dexter reassured me with his characteristic cool. "It's just a hassle. Look at it like an IRS audit."

"The IRS doesn't lead off with a subpoena, do they?" I asked. I had never been audited. Aside from my patient, the vintage shoplifter, I had had almost no dealings whatsoever with the law, so this was alien territory for me. I didn't even have a lawyer.

"We'll get you one," Dexter said, in his take-charge mode. "When you show them you won't roll over, they'll fold. They're bullies, picking on a sick man. That's chickenshit," he snarled, his cowboy drawl coming out, along with his don't-tread-on-me pioneer pluck. "Just don't worry. You've been doing Nate n' Al's great. Keep your eye on the ball. Do your surgery. That's what the good Lord put you here to do, not to lick the balls of those mangy dogs. Don't let this eat you alive. Do you realize what this could do to your immune system?"

There was something distinctly evangelical about Dexter, and not just his belief, unusual in a lettered man of science, in the mind-body connection, the healing power of positive thinking. It certainly wasn't in my Bronx Science mindset, but I knew better than to dismiss anything Dexter was fervent about. Thus I tried to be more spiritual in dealing with my lymphoma, tried not to think of the hard science, because, according to the charts, my odds were bleak. Yet, by listening to Dexter, by taking hope in his hope, I was feeling better. Until now.

Dexter gave me some background on what was behind the invasion of the G-men. An ardent Republican, a defender of laissez-faire capitalism, self-determinism, and state's rights, and an enemy of Big Government, Dexter blamed our current plight on Bill Clinton and the Democrats. Unable to ram through his National Health initiative, Clinton got as a consolation prize something called The Health Insurance Portability and Accountability Act of 1996, also know as the Kennedy-Kassebaum Bill, after Senate sponsors Ted Kennedy and Nancy Kassebaum. Although theoretically designed to make it easier for small businesses to buy health insurance for their employees and for laid-off individuals to acquire coverage, which any doctor would have applauded, there were so many loopholes that favored insurance companies that nothing really changed. What it did add was a new criminal statute for health care fraud that made it easier for the Justice and Health and Human Services departments to go after Medicare and Medicaid fraud.

The FBI was simply flexing its new muscles. "You give a dog false teeth, it's still going to try and bite you, even if they don't work," Dexter said, using an old farm analogy. He noted that the real victims of the new bill would be poor people, who in the end would be denied even more services. The beneficiary, he railed, was Big Insurance, which could squirm out of paying claims and make life a bureaucratic nightmare for paperwork-inundated physicians. "They want to make a federal case about it," Dexter said. "Well, bring it on! It's business, Alvin. It's just business."

I hated business, big and small. The clerical side of medicine seemed to me an invasion of the sanctity of practice, of healing the sick. It took a noble calling off its pedestal. I was so grateful that Karen did all my billing and insurance forms and saved me the clerical details. And I was grateful that Dexter had taken over all the billing for my work at the center and sent me a check when it was all done. So what that I paid him 30 percent for the privilege. Other doctors thought this was Shylockian, if not extortionate. I thought it was worth it, a small price to pay to avoid the soul-deadening drudgery of the endless red tape. I saw myself as a Dickens character—the heroic Dr. Manette in *A Tale of Two Cities*, not the drone clerk Bob Cratchit in *A Christmas Carol*. But now I worried that my aversion was a form of negligence.

"Do you read your tax return?" Dexter asked. "Hell, no. Who can read it? Your CPA can barely read it. You sign it and you send your check. If your number comes up, you deal with it. Alvin, it's just an audit, and they won't get a cent."

"But they're talking about prison, Dexter."

"What the hell do you want Feds to talk about? Liposuction? Blepharoplasty? It makes them feel big, but it's hot air. Insurance is trying to turn the Feds into its bill collectors. You know how far bill collectors get when you tell them to fuck off. Same with these flatfoots."

For all Dexter's swagger and certainty, I was still a worrier. Yes, he could sell Manhattan to the Indians. He had even sold Karen, the world's toughest customer, on plastic surgery, albeit a minor procedure. Karen was a terrible hypochondriac, in the cutest way. That was one of the reasons she married me, I think, to have a doctor permanently on call to assure her she wasn't dying of cancer or some other dreaded disease. To her, every ache was a symptom of some major malady. Talk about leaping to conclusions. But for me, it was a lover's leap. Most medical students are the same way. Once they start learning about diseases, they automatically think they have them. But there isn't enough time to obsess about them, so they get over it.

Karen could put on the bravest, coolest face for my patients and assure them of the safety of everything. But when it came to herself, the idea of anesthesia, of scalpels, of blood was the stuff of nightmares and horror movies. Nevertheless, it took Dexter all of five minutes to get her to undergo a new CO2 laser procedure he had pioneered to soften the vertical age lines emanating from her upper lip, and then to give her silicone lip injections. "You're a beautiful lady with beautiful lips," he had told her. "This will only enhance them." If I had said the same words, Karen would have laughed, or cringed. I guess when Gary Cooper talked, people listened.

But Dexter's circle-the-wagons pep talk wasn't allaying my fears. So we kept walking around those expensive blocks, those blocks whose residents probably had all had some kind of plastic surgery, and who aspired to be worked on one day by the great Dexter Farnham, and maybe some other day, by the great Alvin Reiter. We kept walking and talking.

The whole thing started, Dexter said, when he fired a longtime secretary named Marta. Extremely fat and depressed from seeing all the sleek female patients, Marta was always nagging Dexter to do liposuction on her. But he steadfastly refused, telling Marta her problems were purely psychological. He was convinced she would eat the fat right back. She became fatter than ever and so testy and miserable that Dexter had to let her go. In return, she went to the government and claimed that Dexter, and all the many doctors who worked under him at the center, were making their fortunes by operating on poor Mexicans, charging their medical insurance for fancy cosmetic surgeries only affordable to the rich. Marta was a rat, providing just the kind of cheese the government was looking for.

There had recently been a notorious local case in which a dozen Vietnamese women who worked in the same Atlanta fabric factory had been found to have had nose jobs in Los Angeles to address breathing problems caused by deviated septums, and all had made claims to Prudential Insurance. The Pru's fraud men got curious as to why these women didn't have the work done in Atlanta, where there were plenty of reputable plastic surgeons. The answer, the federal investigators would later charge, was that the women didn't get nasal surgeries at all, but rather rhinoplasties, breast implants, tummy tucks, and "Westernizing" eyelid shaping, all purely "cosmetic" procedures, none of which were covered by their Pru policies. The Feds were claiming that local LA doctors, mostly of Vietnamese origin, were paying these and other Vietnamese women, hooked by ads in Vietnamese newspapers around the country, to fly to sunny LA, stay in a nice hotel, and have "free" plastic surgery, with a trip to Disneyland thrown in for good measure.

The Pru was being suckered, and Big Insurance liked throwing the punches, not taking them. A federal medical dragnet was going on in Southern California, trying to snare more crooked doctors. What could be a brighter feather in the government's cap than nailing a bunch of glamorous Ivy League Beverly Hills surgeons to the stars. It was the stuff law enforcement careers could be made of. It was also the stuff of financial reward for ambitious whistle-blowers, which Dexter surmised was the lure to always cashed-strapped Marta, who spent her generous salary on expensive Rodeo Drive clothes she was always a size too big to wear. All was fair in love and plastic surgery, which had become a competitive war zone, and where *schadenfraude*, or delight at another's downfall, had become as prevalent as in the film business.

The Beverwil Center was a sitting target, as well as a prime one. Unlike hospitals, there was a laxity of record keeping in outpatient clinics. Hospitals have elaborate systems of checks and balances in the documentation of hours. Operating rooms maintain a very tight schedule, and every minute was accounted for. But in outpatient centers, it was easy to fudge that accounting. Hence there was a loophole in the system, and some doctors drove trucks through it, billing $20,000 for a multi-hour complex hernia repair while actually only doing a one-hour $3,500 simple tummy tuck.

"That's outrageous," Dexter said disgustedly. "But that's the kind of junk they're going to try to pin on us. It's so extreme they're going to get laughed out of court."

The idea of being in court, laughing or crying, didn't sit well with me. But whatever boat I was in, I was glad Dexter was my captain. He was too big a man, too great a man for petty crime, or even grand larceny. Yet when Dexter left me, telling me not to worry and to "take one day at a time," I realized he was not without his own flaws, flaws his charisma and surgical genius led everyone who worked for him to overlook. That one-day-at-a-time line was program-speak, the lingo of the twelve-step programs that everyone in Beverly Hills seemed to be part of, at least at some point in their glittering lives. Dexter was in Narcotics Anonymous. Prescription drugs could be a powerful temptation for surgeons, who had easy access to them.

Dexter had fallen, before I ever met him, but he had risen, and he would atone for the rest of his life by going to NA meetings every week and to church every Sunday. In one way, the fact that he was a reformed, God-fearing addict made him an unlikely candidate to be involved in any criminal activity. But, in another way, Beverly Hills doctors, as I had learned, were capable of the biggest surprises, and I began to fret over whether hitching my wagon to Dexter's star might now provide a disastrous ride.

I didn't meet Dexter until I had been in Beverly Hills for over a decade, in 1988. Even though it was a small town, and a small world, there wasn't a community of surgeons, or plastic surgeons, where we would be introduced and get to know each other. Then again, there had been nothing communal, or particularly collegial, about the medical educational experience, so I never expected to be inducted into some chummy secret society where my fellow doctors all wore ties with the same coat of arms.

I was also surprised to see how much money could enter the medical equation. Dr. John Lipton, my first boss, having acquired the glamorous client list of throat-doctor-to-the-stars Henry Rubin, seemed quite shameless in his greed. His was a case of foolish overreach: celebrity and millionaire patients are supersensitive to exploitation. They left in droves when Dr. Lipton tried to talk them into totally unnecessary surgeries or procedures. "Deviated septum" was the seemingly universal diagnosis, and surgery was the recommended treatment. Most of his patients did not have deviated septums, and if they did, they did not need surgery. They knew they were being hoodwinked, and they wouldn't tolerate it. Of course, there was a great deal more money in operating on people than in taking wax out of their ears or sending them down to the pharmacy with a Sudafed prescription. So the patients fled, and Dr. Lipton went to Texas, where he planned to make a fortune in real estate. His departure was undoubtedly influenced by the offer I made to buy the Beverly Hills practice and office lease. I very much wanted to dissociate myself from his unscrupulous behavior, and buying his practice seemed the best way to accomplish this.

This time period was the beginning of what would become an ongoing battle between the general plastic surgeons and the ENT doctors. Understanding this battle will be easier if I clarify what ENT doctors do. People go to ENTs when they have a cold, sore throat, or the flu. An ENT will also treat cancers of the jaw, mouth, throat, and sinuses, as well as any type of malignancy in the head and neck region. ENTs also treat salivary gland problems, do ear surgeries, and remove tonsils. Another kind of ENT might specialize in facial trauma and attendant reconstructive surgery.

Finally, there are the ENTs who see little of the traditional cough and cold business but specialize more in facial plastic surgery, including rhinoplasties, blepharoplasties, otoplasties (ear work), facelifts, and facial implants. As part of his training, an ENT doctor spends four years working on the face and every aspect of it and is thus extremely qualified to do facial plastic surgery. As this became the most lucrative branch of the field, more and more doctors headed in that direction, especially in Beverly Hills.

The history of cosmetic rhinoplasty is closely bound to that of nasal reconstruction. Because of the nose's physical location, it has been regarded as a direct avenue to the brain, man's source of intelligence and spirituality. The nose has been used as a powerful metaphor for a man's character and behavior as seen in culture from Cyrano to Pinocchio. Even Sigmund Freud thought that surgical alterations of the nose could critically influence the mental health of the individual. Although reconstructive rhinoplasty had its roots in ancient India, the celebrity nose job, which had become a symbol of Beverly Hills medicine, had begun in New York in 1923, when Fanny Brice, the star of the Ziegfeld Follies and subject of the Barbra Streisand films *Funny Girl* and *Funny Lady*, had her nose "bobbed" using the hairstyle parlance of the flapper era. The reduction was front page news, the subject of both ridicule and fascination. The Algonquin wit Dorothy Parker quipped that Ms. Brice "had cut off her nose to spite her race." *The New York Times* noted that the public's interest was so high that "one might think it was the greatest engineering feat since the building of the Panama Canal." The man who did Brice's surgery, Harry Schireson, America's first "star" plastic surgeon, was later disgraced and became known as the "King of Quacks."

Any doctor who was interested in this still new field, as I was, couldn't help but be familiar with Schireson's cautionary tale. A Russian immigrant, Schireson grew up on New York's Lower East Side, as did my grandparents. He worked as a drugstore clerk while trying to get an education at a series of geographically diverse but increasingly dubious and unaccredited institutions, culminating in a degree from a diploma mill called the Kansas City College of Medicine and Surgery. He somehow got medical licenses in several states, though not in New York, where he performed Brice's nose job in her apartment in the Ritz Tower on Park Avenue. Schireson may not have been a great doctor, or even a real doctor, but he was a great self-promoter. He got his front-page patients through alliances with the powerful press agents who put those clients on the front pages. Not long after the surgery that made America nose-conscious, Brice's press agent sued Schireson for reneging on the 25 percent commission Schireson had promised him.

Much of Schireson's professional life was spent in court. He later sued a famous British actress, Lady Diana Manners, and her titled mother, the Duchess of Rutland, for failing to pay for the facelifts he had done on both of them. He was sued by another showgirl who had to have both legs amputated after Schireson tried to "reshape" them, resulting in gangrene. Although he ended up going to federal prison for several years, Schireson remained famous, and published a huge bestseller on plastic surgery, *As Others See You*, in 1938. He kept on "doing" the vain, rich, and famous, until his last remaining medical license, in Pennsylvania, was revoked in 1947. He died two years later.

Plastic surgery stayed in the closet for decades, not just because of the scandals and quackery of "doctors" like Harry Schireson, but mainly because no one wanted to admit their beauty was not a gift from God. This attitude went back centuries. Aulus Cornelius Celsus described amazing details in first century Greece and Italy about operations on the nose, lips, and eyelids. In the sixteenth century, Gaspare Tagliacozzi of Bologna became known as the father of modern plastic surgery because of his remarkably enduring techniques of facial reconstruction on victims of the duels and wars of the Renaissance. Tagliacozzi said

Alvin Reiter, MD

that "reconstruction is not performed to please the eye but rather to cheer the spirit of the one afflicted." He had to fight major battles with the Catholic Church, which held that deformities of birth and accident were "the will of God" and must not be tampered with. After his death, Tagliacozzi's soul was damned by the Church and his body was exhumed from its Catholic cemetery and reinterred in a potter's field.

For several hundred years, this blasphemous practice of plastic surgery was suppressed and forgotten, until it was reintroduced in the late eighteenth century in the medical centers of Italy, England, France, and Germany. The first nasal reconstruction was done in Rochester, New York, in 1897, by Dr. John Orlando Roe, and a year later in Berlin by Dr. Jacques Joseph, a protean surgeon who is considered the most important pioneer of present day rhinoplasty. His textbook, *Nasen Plastik*, is still the basic text for modern plastic surgery of the nose.

With the advent of the Boeing 707 plane in the 1960s, a social group known as the "jet set" came into being, the coolest people on earth. Dr. Ivo Pitanguy, a Brazilian plastic surgeon with an apartment in Paris and a ski chalet in Gstaad, was a charter member of this international group. He began making contacts and convincing the beauties of the world that he could make them more beautiful, or at least keep them beautiful longer.

Soon "flying down to Rio" no longer evoked the Astaire-Rogers musical; instead it became code for going to the Pitanguy Clinic for "some work." Though the Brazilian doctor was totally discreet, rumors abounded that goddesses like Brigitte Bardot, Catherine Deneuve, Sophia Loren, Gina Lollobrigida, Melina Mercouri, Candice Bergen, and Marisa Berenson, not to mention world royalty from the Duchess of Windsor to the Empress of Iran, had made the beauty trip to the tropics. Pitanguy was written up in big stories in *Vogue* and the *New York Times*, and many other places. Even I, as a lowly student riding the subway to my education, was aware of his reputation and glamour. The public, always fascinated with the special privileges of movie stars, concluded that if plastic surgery was good for them, it was good for them too. The seeds were thus planted for the birth of a boom.

Once the shame factor was removed, it was only natural that Beverly Hills, home to the stars, would become the fertile crescent of plastic surgery. After all, why fly off into the sunset when you could stay right on Sunset Boulevard? Women who went "on holiday" in Brazil and came back looking younger than ever weren't fooling anyone. Doctors in what would become the 90210 zip code began sharpening their knives.

When I arrived, the ruler of the field in Beverly Hills was a man named Franklyn Ashley. Like so many surgeons and the stars they treated, Ashley was a dominant, decisive character. Unlike other surgeons, but not unusual for Beverly Hills doctors, Ashley had a social life. He actually took vacations. His hobby was big game hunting, and his office was festooned with stuffed lion heads and elephant tusks and real zebra skin couches. His best friend was John Wayne, upon whom he reportedly did a facelift. It wasn't all he-man stuff, though. He was also pals with Fred Astaire, who saw no need to fly down to Rio when he was ready for his facelift. And he reconstructed Ann Margaret when she fell off a stage into an orchestra pit in a Lake Tahoe casino. But the star who put Ashley in the public eye was anything but a beauty queen. It was comedienne Phyllis Diller, whose self-deprecation about her appearance was such a part of her act that she had nothing to lose by turning her surgery into a major subject of humor on the *Tonight Show* and anywhere else in the media that she could get a laugh.

Ashley became the first brand-name plastic surgeon. Before him, plastic surgery in Beverly Hills had been largely a backstreet affair. An old-timer I met named Michael Gurdin had done Marilyn Monroe's chin and Clark Gable's ears, among many other celebrity features, yet if either of them ever saw him in public, they would cross the street or leave a restaurant to avoid him, for fear of exposure. Other stars simply went far away, to Rio or New York, to avoid scrutiny. Both Gary Cooper and Joan Crawford had their facelifts done by the Park Avenue surgeon, John Marquis Converse, who later married Cooper's widow, Rocky.

In the late 70s, when I arrived in town, Franklyn Ashley, the reigning king of plastic surgery, was nearing retirement, demand was skyrocketing, and all my fellow doctors wanted a piece of this sweetest of pies. All I wanted to do was get started. I thus had to accept removing earwax and draining sinuses as my immediate lot in my new life. I was hardly a networker, but I took John Lipton's advice and introduced myself to doctors in our building and block of Roxbury, and along the parallel doctors' row of Bedford. That's how I met the famous Rex Kennamer. I also met Ed Kantor, who had our biggest rival celebrity ENT practice. He seemed like a TV doctor, like Robert Young, while his young associate, Joe Sugarman, who wore cowboy boots and jeans, looked like a rock star. If that was what it would take to draw famous clients, I was doomed.

Luckily we had plenty of clients, famous, rich, and just folks, and I was happy to treat them all. Just seeing the plaque on the oak door— ALVIN REITER, MD—was reward enough. I especially liked the Roxbury office because of its 1940s feel. I could imagine Lana Turner and Rita Hayworth coming down the halls. Our equipment was quite old fashioned, which was part of the charm. We had a glass booth where the staff audiologist did hearing tests. As much as I liked the place, I didn't place my diplomas on the walls of Lipton's office, which I would use to consult with patients. I was very much the outsider, and somehow I didn't feel of the place, which was natural, because I was not.

At lunch I would walk the streets of Beverly Hills and look at all the stars who called this town home. I saw the whole Rat Pack— Frank Sinatra, Dean Martin, Peter Lawford, Sammy Davis Jr., Shirley MacLaine—all just walking around. I saw James Stewart, Joseph Cotten, poor fat Orson Welles, poor old Martha Raye, poor, sick Barbara Hutton (well, she wasn't really poor). I saw everybody, just taking a walk, which was pretty thrilling. For lunch, I ate at this little coffee shop that was part of the Mickey Fine Pharmacy, which was to doctors what Nate'n Al's was to comedians. The name made me think of a Mickey Finn, the knock-out drink, but there was nothing soporific about this bustling nerve center of the medical golden triangle. The counter was a good place to meet other doctors, who ate, if at all, on the fly. It was less intimidating than calling on them in their offices, like a drug company sales rep. Actually I got more referrals from the nice pharmacist at Mickey Fine's, who was from the Bronx, than from the doctors.

It was hard to get patients. I thought all of Henry Rubin's stars would come our way, but word got out that John Lipton was trying to trade them all up to nasal reconstruction. Soon it seemed that all of Rubin's patients had been captured by Kantor and Sugarman. Maybe I needed some cowboy boots after all. Henry Rubin soon took his name off our door. He had stopped paying for malpractice insurance and was worried that if John or I did something wrong he would be potentially liable for our mistakes. That was a nice vote of no confidence, but this was the dawn of the litigation era, and the last thing a doctor wanted was to be spending his time with lawyers. In any event, I was totally turned off by Lipton's aggressive medical self-marketing and began thinking about ways to disassociate myself from him.

I tried to network by meeting other doctors, who I hoped would refer patients to me. One prominent practitioner invited me to lunch at Hillcrest Country Club, which was Jewish Valhalla. It had its own oil well on the golf course and cost a fortune to join, if you could pass the board. I saw Groucho Marx, George Jessel, Milton Berle, and George Burns all sitting together at what the doctor told me was "the comics' table." I also saw Sammy Davis Jr., who was the club's token black member, but, then again, Sammy was Jewish. I had visions of the doctor becoming my friend and sponsoring me for membership. I would learn golf, tell jokes, be invited to the comics' table, and charm my way into a celebrity practice. My bubble was quickly burst when the doctor hit me up the entire lunch for a big donation to the State of Israel. In my tenuous financial state, I was in no position to donate to anything, and as soon as the doctor saw that, he knew I was not "his people." That was the end of what I thought might be the beginning of a beautiful friendship. He never sent me a patient, and I never saw him again.

One way I built my practice was through being on the staff of numerous area hospitals, which necessitated a lot of emergency room night calls, but it came with the turf. I hated the violence that usually brought the people in, but the opportunity to help these victims was gratifying. And once you had operated on someone and saved a life, there was no greater love between doctor and patient, and the referrals began to flood in.

But before they did, John Lipton decided he didn't have enough business to warrant maintaining two offices. In 1978, he decided to consolidate in his Century City facility, which had its own operating room. He was going to close the Roxbury office. Elaine, who had confidence in my ability to be out on my own, pushed me to buy the practice from him. Here was my chance to break with Lipton. I didn't need another partner, she insisted. She came with me to City National Bank and co-signed a $50,000 loan—$30,000 to buy the practice, or what was left of it, and $20,000 to survive on for the next year. Her business timing was impeccable. Soon after signing the papers, the patients I never thought would materialize began making appointments.

If only our romantic timing had been as good. Elaine was constantly depressed, not over the cultural wasteland that she assumed Los Angeles would be (but actually was not), but over her dislike of the practice of medicine. The more she did it, the less she liked it. Her heart was that of an artist, and she couldn't find any artistry in her family practice at Kaiser. The "Kaiser way" of seeing a patient every six minutes was inhuman in her eyes. She wasn't an assembly line doctor. She loved medicine, and took the Hippocratic oath seriously. She had a strong moral and religious background, and charity and kindness were second nature to her. She was from a blue-collar family and had worked hard to become a doctor, but this just wasn't the way she had seen herself developing.

She was a great pianist, a great violinist, a great embroiderer. Those delicate hands of hers were made for surgery, not for Kaiser, which was a huge medical factory. I suggested that she try to find a family doctor near me she could partner with, something approximating a small town practice. But it didn't matter anymore to Elaine where she practiced, or with whom. Kaiser had turned her against the medical profession. Despite all my emergency room calls, I wasn't working the kamikaze schedule I had during my training. I had a bit of time for dinners, for walks, for the Hollywood Bowl. We had bought a nice little house in Brentwood, a lovely, quiet, leafy place, perfect for two struggling yuppies.

I had never thought about other women as long as Elaine and I were married. She was the first love of my life. We had gone through our medical education together, and while that was an intense bond, I'm not sure how romantic it actually was. I was a fairly square straight arrow who never imagined straying.

I had a pretty receptionist named Shawn. It sounds sexist, or looksist, but if you were in the plastic surgery business, or wanted to be in it, you had to lead with an ace. First impressions were lasting, and every office I visited had a cover girl-type receptionist. Given that Hollywood was a magnet for every beauty queen from every town in the country, and given how unlikely it was for any of them to realize their dreams of stardom, there was a huge talent pool of potential receptionists. So Lipton had Shawn, whom I kept after buying out the Roxbury office.

Shawn had a lot of pretty friends. One of them, a Minnesota blond dairy queen named Brigid, who worked as a speech therapist until her celluloid ship came in, had been a patient of Lipton's. He was treating her for a sinus infection, and one of the tenets of such treatment is to drain the sinuses and shrink the swollen nasal mucosa in the process. Despite its lurid images and associations with the Medellin Cartel, cocaine is a mainstay of ENT treatment. It works wonderfully to shrink swollen mucosa as well as to anaesthetize the nose. However, as with all drugs, there are toxic levels. One Friday afternoon, after Lipton had gone to play golf in Palm Springs, Brigid realized the cocaine Lipton had used to drain her sinuses earlier that day was flipping her out.

So I came to the rescue, meeting her at the office and staying with her for eight hours until she came down. I was worried she might die of a heart attack, and also, to a lesser extent, that Lipton's practice would be destroyed by a major malpractice lawsuit, not to mention cocaine scandal that could destroy, by association, my own practice before it had even begun. But she pulled through, and I never saw her as a patient, though she continued to see Lipton, despite his almost killing her to drain her sinuses. She would always say hi to me in the office, and after Lipton left, she still would drop by to visit Shawn and go for after-work cocktails. One day Shawn blushingly told me Brigid had a crush on me, the man who saved her life. Because in my sheltered medical foxhole I hadn't heard that kind of thing before, I found it highly flattering.

I began having longer and longer chats with Brigid when she would come by to pick up Shawn and go to the Beverly Wilshire or the Polo Lounge for drinks at the close of the day. Brigid's father had been a north woods country doctor, and for some inexplicable reason she seemed to find me fascinating. In any event, to make a sad story short, her flattery got her everywhere, most specifically my Brentwood abode, while Elaine had taken a week off to visit her family in Connecticut. We had gone for a relaxing walk on the Venice canals, and then Brigid insisted on coming home and making me a Mexican dinner, a new skill she wanted to try out on me. The kitchen was virgin territory, as neither Elaine nor I ever cooked. There were a lot of laughs when it turned out we had nothing to cook with, no spices, no napkins. One margarita led to another.

When Elaine returned she found a birth control pill wrapper on the floor under the bed. I immediately told her the truth. I was sorry. It had never happened before, but I knew I couldn't guarantee that it wouldn't happen again. I moved out of the bedroom and slept on the couch until we could sort out our feelings. Elaine figured things out fast. She wanted to stay married. She was so anaesthetized to our life as it was that she didn't even get that upset. She never suggested couples therapy, or any psychological intervention. She was willing to sweep it all under the rug.

But I wasn't. Within a month, I rented a small apartment at the Casa Granada complex on Barrington Avenue in Brentwood and moved out. Elaine never called me. I never called her. I got a lawyer. Then Elaine got a lawyer. It was totally amicable. It was totally sad. We never sat down to have a postmortem about what went wrong. We just dissolved as a couple. We stopped seeing each other. I gave Elaine the Brentwood house without a fight. I would have given her everything. I was impressed by my divorce lawyer, who was anything but a shark. She is your wife, after all, he said. Thus when I gladly gave Elaine the house the lawyer called it "menschy," but I called it a combination of guilt and conflict avoidance. I never saw Brigid again. I just went back to work.

In the middle of my marital Sturm und Drang, on my way to an emergency call to Santa Monica Hospital, a big van plowed into me at the corner of Sunset and Barrington. I wasn't hurt, but my trusty old Plymouth Scamp was totaled. I was impressed that the police car on the scene put on its siren and rushed me to the hospital, not for my injuries, which were negligible, but so that I could perform my surgery. The next day I went out to buy a new car. I was going to buy a big Cadillac, because Cadillacs seemed safe, but then Shawn scolded me about how uncool it would be to drive a Cadillac. So I went to the opposite extreme and looked at a Ferrari. The salesman, a Rudolf Valentino look-alike who wore a slick Italian suit and reeked of alcohol, ranted on about how the Ferrari would change me life, and then reeled off a list of other doctor clients. His closing pitch was, "Hey, man, if you want to be a plastic surgeon, you gotta drive this mother."

I fled to the Mercedes dealer, which seemed to offer the right compromise between substance and flash. The salesman there, a sober type, said he had only three words for me. "DO IT NOW!" So I did, purchasing a red 450SL convertible. I must have been out of my mind with the inner turmoil over the dissolution of my marriage, my starting my own practice, and my first affair bursting forth. I suddenly wanted to mourn the life I was leaving behind. I drove the Mercedes to the auto graveyard. I got out and wandered through the wreckage until I found my poor crumpled Scamp. I pried open the door and climbed in. I thought about growing up in the Bronx, about Elaine, about med school, about everything. And then, all alone in the Scamp, where no one could see me, I broke down and cried.

Chapter Four

BEDFELLAS

To recover from what amounted to my loss of innocence, I threw myself into my work with a fervor reminiscent of my residency days. In the process, I started making some doctor friends. I met a fellow recent bachelor, Tim Harold, an ENT surgeon who looked a lot like Robert Redford. Tim drove a British racing green Aston Martin, like the one in *Goldfinger*, and had a big boat in the marina, like those owned by James Bond villains, and packed with nearly as many bikini-clad girls. Tim let me do facelifts with him, and also taught me the ropes in the hot new field of hair transplantation, which I disliked doing at the time because the results looked so unnatural. (It's come a long way since then.)

My brother's rich wife, Suzyn, introduced me to the husband of one of her girlhood friends, Rod Baxter, who was with the power fiefdom of Greene and Roberts, the nose job cartel. He broke up with them when he refused to do their "ghost surgeries." Like Hollywood screenwriters, Beverly Hills plastic surgeons wanted credit for their masterpieces. Money wasn't enough, and the egos of Greene and Roberts were too big to allow any credit to filter downward. So without money in the bank, Rod, a New Yorker with a residency at Mt. Sinai to his credit, went off on his own. He would often ask me to join him in challenging operative situations.

Rod had offices at 9201 Sunset, which was full of powerful Hollywood law firms and casting agencies. The office belonged to another face man of a plastic surgeon named Mark Cranston, who in his twenties had been "the Brylcreem Man" on billboards all over the country. Just as it was essential for a plastic surgeon to have great-looking receptionists and nurses, being great-looking himself could only seal the deal for a wavering patient, especially a female one. Cranston, who had one of the first state-of-the-art operating rooms right in his office suite, was also a trailblazer: he starred in his own cable TV show on plastic surgery. Although very few homes nationwide had cable at that point, most homes in the Beverly Hills area did, and Mark profited mightily from the media exposure of his chiseled features and pomaded hair. For a long while, his girlfriend was the TV star Loretta Swit of *MASH*, and the combination of Mr. Brylcreem and Hot Lips Houlihan captured the imagination of media-obsessed potential patients.

Being around such fast-lane doctors made it inevitable that I would meet some fast-lane women. Being single, and feeling liberated, I was open to socializing. In those days, before the dawn of sexual harassment, it was perfectly natural for doctors to date their patients. Where else was a busy doctor going to meet people? A doctor's social life was either his nurses or his patients. I would meet people in strange ways. The celebrity realtor Stan Herman (who was married to TV star Linda Evans), whom I had met when Elaine and I went house hunting, referred a stunning blonde named Vanessa, heiress of a tractor fortune in Nebraska, for a second opinion after another ENT had told her she needed surgery for a fractured cheekbone she suffered in an accident in her Rolls Royce. Since hers was a non-displaced fracture, I recommended that she leave it alone. Having dreaded the prospect of surgery, she was so grateful and relieved that she invited me to lunch at the Bistro Garden, a haunt of Nancy Reagan and the Beverly Hills wives of her husband's kitchen cabinet, Betsy Bloomingdale and company.

Stan Herman seemed to know only rich beautiful women to whom he could sell multi million dollar homes. Some were starlets and showgirls who had married, and divorced, very well; others, like Vanessa, were from rich families. Vanessa automatically assumed that if Stan Herman recommended me, I must have done plastic surgery on Linda Evans and Bo Derek and Herman's other high-profile love interests. Because doctors can never reveal the identities of their patients, I chose to be sphinxlike, neither confirming nor denying, as the CIA says to all media requests, and let Vanessa's imagination run wild, which it did. A young woman in her early thirties, Vanessa had mansions both in Bel Air and Montecito, the Bel Air of Santa Barbara, and I enjoyed riding up the coast in her Rolls convertible. As it turned out, Vanessa had a deeply jealous and very large brute of a boyfriend who showed up at my apartment late one night stalking her. I was lucky she wasn't there, but I still had to call the police. That romance was over in a flash.

I began dating two "trophy" women, Melissa, the daughter of a legendary Hollywood movie star, and Alexis, the daughter of a billionaire who owned one of the nation's most successful sports franchises. I guess being a single Beverly Hills plastic surgeon made me a highly eligible bachelor, but for all that and the Mercedes convertible, I never saw myself as more than a Bronx Science subway scholar. In any event, I was taken to glamorous parties and glittering events, although they rarely yielded referrals, which again were more likely to come through the likes of the pharmacist at Mickey Fine or my Mercedes mechanic, real people as opposed to the high and mighty.

Strangely enough, in a city full of Jewish girls, I never met any of them. And then Karen Braun appeared. Karen's family had been patients of Henry Rubin for decades, and they were one of the few families who didn't decamp for the Kantor office when Henry retired. I had met her father first. Bob Braun owned Vendome, a high-end chain of liquor stores that catered to the Chasen's crowd. Bob was a tall, sporty tennis player, and something of a vain playboy, which I discovered when he asked me to give him a hair transplant, which I did with my Redfordian colleague Tim Harold.

I liked Bob and his wife, Mimi, a true looker in her youth and once the personal secretary to studio chief Jack Warner, from whom Bob had wooed her away. Mimi had lots of colds and sinus problems, and I finally came to understand the line from the Rogers and Hart song "The Lady is a Tramp," "She hates California, it's cold and it's damp," which Sinatra had sung so often. Despite its image of eternal sunshine, California, even Southern California, could be wet and rainy and as good an incubator of respiratory illness as the Bronx.

Bob and Mimi's daughter, Gail, was a frequent patient. She was married to a very attractive and dynamic up-and-coming lawyer in a big Century City firm. I treated her five-year-old daughter. Gail had the mysterious complaint that the girl's nose "smelled." I quickly solved the mystery by finding a decomposing green pea up her nostril. I took a nasal instrument called a canula, connected it to a suction machine, and within twenty minutes had extracted the pea from the princess. Gail thought I was a genius; when I refused to charge her, she thought I was a saint.

That set the stage for my first appointment with Karen, the younger sister who was as lovely and as charming as Gail. It was 1978, and Karen was an elementary school teacher in a tough Latino neighborhood in

East Los Angeles. For some reason I felt immediately protective of her. Although she was 31, she seemed very girlish. She had huge expressive eyes, like my mother's, which I had called "cherry eyes" as a kid. Karen's were similar. Her nose was perfect, one that even a super-critic like myself could have used as a model for what a nose could aspire to. Karen had come in for me to check out her ears so she could be certified for a scuba diving course she was taking. Nice Jewish girls don't scuba dive, I thought to myself.

When I examined Karen's ears I was intoxicated by the scent of her perfume. I had an instant crush. I remember doing something far beyond the canons of ethics. I looked up Karen's address and drove by her house, where she still lived with her parents. It wasn't grand luxe Beverly Hills but the far more bourgeois Beverlywood, south of Pico Boulevard, definitely the wrong side of the tracks in this status-crazy community. Still, it was a lovely house with a fine garden and tall deciduous trees that reminded me of the East. I whistled "On the Street where You Live" to myself: "I have often walked down this street before. But the pavement always stayed beneath my feet before. All at once am I several stories high, knowing I'm on the street where you live." I couldn't have cared less if the street had been in Watts. I drove up and down the block ten times, hoping that Karen would step out into an "accidental" encounter. Typically for LA, I didn't see a soul in the street. This isolation allowed me to indulge in my temporary insanity, a romantic moment in a life without any.

I didn't see Karen again for another year. By then I had split with Elaine and was dating bombshells and heiresses. Yet the minute I saw Karen again, for an earache, I was riveted. She was the perfect Jewish girlfriend I had never had. My mother would adore her. Once a dedicated teacher, Karen had been mugged at her elementary school by a non-student serially preying on both faculty and students. Much as I admired Karen for her commitment to teaching the under-privileged, I couldn't blame her for being scared out of her wits. She had wanted to teach in the ghetto, where fine, dedicated teachers were scarce, and she found out the cause of the scarcity the hard way.

Now she had swung to the other extreme, gotten a real estate license, and was selling high-end properties for one of Stan Herman's rivals for the silk stocking trade. I made an impulsive decision that I would move out of my bachelor pad into a proper Beverly Hills doctor's house. Karen could be my agent. What I hoped, subconsciously at this point, was that Karen would live there with me. Later on Karen told me that she had suggested to her mother that I was flirting with her. Her mother dismissed the idea, saying to Karen, "You should be so lucky."

Soon Karen and I were having dinners together under the guise of real estate meetings. As much as I liked her, I was juggling those two trophy women and would ask her romantic advice, hiding the fact that the real romance I was feeling was for her. But somehow I suppressed it for a long time, and Karen and I became good friends. I guess it was too soon after divorcing Elaine for me to think of getting married again, and I didn't want to waste Karen's time. She had lots of suitors, all of whom she complained about to me. She complained about everything, she worried about her health, but she did it all in a highly endearing way. She was like a comedienne with, not a death wish, but a death schtick. Whatever she had, it was going to kill her. As her comic foil, I had to joke my way out of her anxiety. Yet for all her "cootie-phobia," as we referred to her aversion to germs, Karen was a terrific athlete, a strong swimmer, skier, and tennis player, like her sportsman father, and anything but a homebody. She got me to go scuba diving with her, and dragged me to the pool at the Beverly Hills YMCA. We would go rent rowboats in Echo Park. We'd ride bikes on the Venice bike path and marvel at the volleyball games at Muscle Beach.

The only thing we wouldn't do was go to restaurants. Karen was obsessed with her weight, and could have been the poster girl for Weight Watchers, the commoner counterpart of spokesperson Sarah Ferguson, Duchess of York. With her passion for all things English, from rose gardens to high tea to Lord Peter Wimsey, Karen, I would joke, was my Duchess of Beverly Hills. It was hard to believe but, as a teenager, Karen had carried more than 200 pounds on her five-foot-five-inch small-boned frame. Her parents sent her to Duke University for its famous rice diet, but she would sneak off campus at night to buy candy bars at convenience stores and chocolate cakes at the Piggly Wiggly supermarket, and she returned home heavier than she had left. The deep pain that Karen experienced from being fat is clear from the letters she wrote to her mother when she was eighteen years old:

Dear Mommy,

I'm so sad. I love you and I don't like to be unhappy and make you unhappy. Why am I so weak? I'm so frightened! I have no confidence in myself. I say I've made up my mind and I'm going to diet—but my mind is so easily unmade. I haven't dieted for a weekend in so long, I could just kill myself!!! It's so ridiculous and disgusting - it's a vicious circle. I've got to diet!!! I've got till June 12th and I'd better make up my mind to lose all I can possibly or die. This afternoon when you said I'm going to be fat and marry a fat man I could have killed myself. But does that stop me?—no!! I still manage to stuff my face!!! I want to be happy so much and the thing that will make me happy will be being thin and I can be thin if I just diet. Why am I denying myself of this?? Why??? I want it so badly!?!?!?!?!? What's worse, I have no self-respect anymore!! I have no will power - no self-discipline!! Oh, I'm so depressed what am I going to do?? I probably gained five pounds this stupid weekend!! I wish there was only Monday to Friday afternoon—no Friday night—to Sunday!!—Then I'd probably cheat on another day. I feel so hopeless and helpless—Is there any hope for me? Mommy, I need you—I'm really scared!! Please love me and don't give up - cause if you don't have confidence then things are really bad. I love you with all my heart and I wish I could please you by doing the one thing that would make you happy.

Love & xxxxxx, Karen

Dear Mom and Dad,

I didn't stay on my diet today and I am mad at myself. But, I'm not depressed. I'm very happy in fact. It has been so beautiful lately, and I feel honored just to be alive. (Like today at school, when it seemed like you could just reach out and touch the mountains.) Weight and school are stupid, stupid things to be depressed about. It's just that lately I've really been thinking about it, and all of a sudden I realize I'm fat, and want to lose weight. Like Daddy said before—you must 1st realize and admit to yourself—that you have a problem, before you can do anything about it. It's hard for me to admit that I am different from my family, that I am one of "those other" people. But I think I'm beginning to. I want to be thin. For a long time, I've just wanted to be on a diet, to be on a diet, but now, all of a sudden, I want to be thin. But, I still can't do anything about it! I hope this hypnosis thing is successful. All of a sudden, I'm really jazzed on it. I love you - and aside from being fat - I am very happy!

Love and xxxx, Karen

Eventually Karen lost weight and kept it under control, holding the line at a svelte 115 pounds, but she knew she had a powerful sugar addiction. She wanted me never to lead her into temptation. Restaurants were her devil.

So I ate out with my other girlfriends. Alexis eventually fell by the wayside, but Melissa stayed the course for years. When Melissa started making marriage noises, she forced me to think seriously about Karen. Until then, Karen was the best pal a guy could have. Meanwhile she found me a beautiful house, also in Brentwood, which was getting more desirable every day, and helped me furnish it. I think it was the only house she ever sold because she couldn't stand the phoniness of being a realtor and missed teaching. She always preferred poor to rich, and real estate, West LA real estate, was a rich person's game.

My parents came to visit me in California for the first time in 1980; before that, I had flown back to New York whenever I had a break. They were incredibly proud of my office, down the hall from Rex Kennamer, whom they had heard of from reading *Photoplay*, the fifties movie magazine that was the *People* of its day. Their fantasy of "my son the doctor" had come true. By that point I was earning more than $100,000 a year, a huge sum at the time. They were happy for me and vastly relieved, I think, because I know they had their doubts about my potential for worldly success.

If my practice was Exhibit A of the good life I was leading, my friend Karen was Exhibit B, the Jewish girl of their dreams. My mother wasn't the pushy sort who would say, "Marry her," but I knew she was relieved Elaine was gone, and she genuinely liked Karen, who was so kind, driving her all over, showing her the sights. My father, meanwhile, found some of his transplanted New York buddies and drank, smoked cigars, played cards, and reminisced about their glory days.

Karen was my dearest friend, male or female. In 1984, after nearly six years of friendship, I was ready for true love. My wild oats had been sewn and I never looked back.

It was another new chapter in my life. The New York chapter had closed earlier that year with the death of my father from stomach cancer at age 73. He and my mother had been out to visit the year before, and he looked frailer than usual. His spirits were high, so I just assumed he was aging. But the cancer struck quickly, and neither parent told me until my father was literally on his deathbed. I think they still saw me as their little boy and tried to shield me from all bad news. I felt awful, thinking that if they'd brought me into the loop, I might have been able to save him. But then I pinched myself; the cancer he had was an inevitable death sentence. Doctors did all they could, that was their duty, their mission, but they were realists when it came to the odds. I was fortunate to have made it to New York to spend my father's last weekend with him. I was at his bedside at the hospital when he died.

When my father died, I wanted my mother to come and live in Los Angeles. I was doing well enough to support her. But I never got the chance to discuss it with her. Soon after my father's funeral, she went into a coma. She was in a New Jersey hospital for months, until she was transferred by state social services to a nursing home. She eventually came out of the coma, but she was never the same as before. Her life force had been drained.

Between flying back and forth to sit by her side, I researched possible Los Angeles nursing homes, but I found them to be a sorry affair, much worse than the one in New Jersey where she had her own room, attentive care, and a serene view over the Hudson. I knew a fair amount about LA senior care from my early days in practice, when I did a circuit of nursing homes to take wax out of patients' ears. Nothing I had seen in LA could come close to where my mother was. I usually found her sitting up in a chair, seemingly alert, and happy to see me. But at other times she was very distant. I'm not sure she always recognized me, but I invariably felt the visits from me and Karen brought her joy. I loved hearing her stories. She was still beautiful, with red hair and big cherry eyes. But I had no idea what those eyes were seeing.

My mother lived until 1992. Karen and I would go to visit her three or four times a year, and once, in 1988, we took Karen's mother as well, for a kind of family reunion. One day I took a break from the home and drove my rental car over the George Washington Bridge to the Bronx. What had happened to the old homestead was nearly as heartbreaking as what had happened to my family. The Bronx was a war zone, those elegant deco apartments turned into burned-out shells, or at best shooting gallery tenements. The day was gray and cold, bleak and grim, like something out of Soviet Russia. I drove to Mt. Hope Place and stared at our old building, once so proud, now a wreck. There was no hope left. I cried for an hour, just sitting there. Then I drove back over the George Washington, said an unheard farewell to my beautiful mother, and flew back to the eternal sunshine of my new California life.

Married life agreed with me, and with my practice. With Karen by my side, I had no distractions whatsoever. Moreover, she was great for business. Having searched for an outlet for her talents that real estate could not provide, Karen took over running my office. Patients adored her, and my billings took off exponentially. I made my first million in 1988, barely ten years after opening my office. I wasn't alone. Beverly

Hills medicine could be tremendously lucrative, and I had what I would call a "normal" practice, not one like Rex Kennamer's, where every patient was rich and/or famous.

But I, too, had plenty of stars. Being an ENT specialist, I got lots of the great singers and Broadway stars who happened to have problems when they were out west doing film or television. Often I had no idea who they were, particularly the rock musicians who sold millions of records to teenage kids. I was a forties guy; any washed up lounge singer from that era would have excited me far more than a glam rocker from the Billboard charts. I also had a lot of screenwriters, playwrights, and book authors, many of whom were Bronx or Brooklyn boys and felt more at home with me than they would with one of my surfer colleagues who seemed too laid back to be serious.

I met many Beverly Hills doctors when I used their operating rooms to do outpatient surgery, which is how I eventually met Dexter Farnham. I was always looking for places to do my surgery, and ended up with some strange bedfellows in the process. I didn't build my own theater because I didn't have room in my office, nor did I want to move out, particularly after Karen inspired me to redecorate it with authentic forties pieces we searched for on weekends at auctions and elegant antique shops on Melrose Place, in LA's super-chic design district. We also created something of a miniature botanical garden, an extension of our home. We did reach a point where we had so much greenery there was barely room for patients.

One of the first surgeons I affiliated with was a man named Harold Brooks, who had a fabulous operating room on Wilshire Boulevard. I eventually learned never to judge a doctor by his operating room, for Brooks was as unreliable as his OR was impeccable. To begin with,

Brooks had a lovely nurse named Treva, who he let do all his breast implant surgeries while the patients were out cold. A compulsive gambler, Brooks would go into his office and bet on sporting events and come out to take all the credit after Treva had neatly sewed the patients completely up, leaving the last few stitches to the doctor.

But that was only the beginning. Brooks also employed a striking Asian woman named Suzy as a "capper," or shill. Suzy was Chinese but had grown up in Saigon; she would go out and round up Vietnamese patients, sell them on the wonders of plastic surgery, and get a bounty of 10 to 20 percent of the surgery bill for every mark she lured in. I learned that most Beverly Hills plastic surgeons retained cappers, one for each ethnic target community: Vietnamese, Chinese, Korean, Japanese, Russian, Persian, Israeli, Hispanic. This was long before the scandals erupted in 1997.

Los Angeles was one of America's chief melting pots, luring immigrants in the hundreds of thousands from all over the world. "Melt" was the word. These newcomers, already hooked on American movies and television before they arrived, wanted to be as American as McDonald's apple turnovers. And they wanted to look American, which meant getting rid of their exotic noses, eyelids, flat chests. Harold Brooks was much more a breast man than a nose man. He wanted me to do all his Vietnamese noses. Not only did he provide the patients, which spared me the dirty work of advertising and the even dirtier work of hiring cappers, neither of which I could defile myself to do, but he paid me more than I would have charged, even minus the fee he deducted for anesthesiology and overhead. I got to do what I loved, which was operate, and Brooks took care of the rest.

How did they afford it, I wondered time after time. "These people have so much money," Brooks would say, exploding the myth of the starving immigrant with the reality of the new, wealthy immigrant.

Of all the immigrant groups, no one was richer than the Persians, most of whom had fled their country after the fall of the Shah in the mid '70s. The Shah's sister came to live in Beverly Hills, as did thousands of her countrymen, all of whom seemed to have made fortunes in Iran and were able to escape the Ayatollah with their money intact. Persians bought a great deal of property in Beverly Hills and Santa Monica, which became known as Isfahan-sur-Mer. Farsi became the majority language at Beverly Hills High School. And the plastic surgery suites of the Golden Triangle were filled with Middle Easterners who thought their wealth would enable them to transform into the likes of Robert Redford and Jane Fonda. This was America, where even the wildest dreams were supposed to come true, especially if you were rich to begin with.

For all their wealth, the Persians, true to their homeland culture, liked to bargain. They wanted all kinds of plastic surgery, but they didn't want to pay for it. That's what this health insurance we have is for, they'd insist. I'd try to explain that health insurance was for health, not vanity, and that purely cosmetic procedures like rhinoplasties were not covered. "Oh, but Dr. So-and-So down the block said he'd take the insurance. Why won't you?" At first I'd call their bluff, sending them to Dr. So-and-So, but it turned out that he was actually taking the insurance.

Medical journals began advertising seminars on "creative billing procedures" that would accommodate the spiraling demand for cosmetic procedures by justifying at least part of the work as a medical necessity. One such instruction course at a national meeting of plastic surgeons was titled "Coding Rhinoplasty and Nasal Reconstruction for Insurance." The brochure read, "Instruction will cover making functional rhinoplasty and nasal reconstruction more rewarding, especially for mixed cosmetic/insurance cases. Diagnostic coding and appeal of insurance claims will be discussed." The august journal *Facial Plastic Times* had a major article on how the problem of payment or any procedure that included a rhinoplasty had been an old and recurring issue. The standard approach was to bill the insurance company for the functional (e.g. nasal obstruction) repair, and the patient for the cosmetic work (nose job). It wasn't only nose jobs. Ptsosis (drooping of the upper eyelid) was often used as the functional justification for billing insurers for cosmetic eyelid reconstruction. The article noted how patients were constantly inveigling doctors "to get my insurance to pay for it" and exhorted doctors to withstand such pressures and "play straight with insurers."

It was indeed like tax laws, wherein sharp tax accountants and clever lawyers found loopholes for their clients. Now doctors were being pressured to push the envelope of medical necessity to avoid losing business. Even I fell prey to this syndrome of looking far harder for breathing difficulties and making more out of deviated septums that I ever had before. I found myself confronted with many more financially hip patients complaining of breathing difficulties and at the same time requesting a change of appearance to their nose. Now no one wanted to avoid surgery, not when it involved looking better, and I began to rethink my old-fashioned take on things.

If Harold Brooks was in the forefront of Asian plastic surgery, another doctor with whom I worked was trying to corner the biggest market of all: the Hispanic one. I had met Goran Porec in 1978 at the Cedars-Sinai emergency room. Goran was Croatian—American by way of Montreal, where he had fled during the Vietnam era to avoid being drafted. He cultivated a suave, unplaceable foreign accent, had a charming French wife who was a genuine antiques dealer, and generally projected the aura of European aristocracy, even though his father actually worked in the stockyards in Chicago.

I later learned that Goran had left Canada under a cloud and gone to Aspen, where he was one of the first plastic surgeons to set up shop in the burgeoning ski resort. He left Aspen under a cloud too. Beverly Hills, I suppose, was the last resort of some scoundrels, the ideal place to reinvent oneself. I found it fascinating that nobody here seemed to care where you went to school, where you had worked before, anything about your past. Nothing mattered except success—present success. In Los Angeles, the past was not prologue but rather something to be erased. Or reconstructed.

The David Begelman case serves as a perfect example. Begelman was the Columbia studio chief accused, and later convicted, of forging and stealing Cliff Robertson's paychecks, among other things. Nobody could believe he had done it. After all, he was a graduate of Yale Law School. It turned out that he had once visited Yale on a Grey Line tour, and that he was a Bronx high school dropout with a daring imagination. Nobody here cared about the truth, only the chutzpah. After doing a brief prison stint for his Columbia crimes, the phony Yale man was forgiven and rewarded by being chosen by his cronies to be head of MGM. Years later, saddled with gambling debts he couldn't lie his way out of, he committed suicide, and all Hollywood wept for him.

And so it was for Goran Porec. No matter what atrocities he may have committed in Montreal and Aspen, Hollywood welcomed him as a surgical genius. He was "modern": he advertised in every imaginable magazine, newspaper insert, and supermarket throwaway. He did infomercials on cable TV, which was then in its infancy. He rented ballrooms in hotels, from the Beverly Hilton to the Airport Hilton, and showed films of himself operating, and endless "Before and After" photos of his patients. He was Doctor 90210 long before TV took over the message. But Goran couldn't have cared less about Hollywood. The real money—movie star money—was to be made not on Sunset Boulevard but on Atlantic Boulevard, the main thoroughfare in East Los Angeles, the Mexican barrio. Horace Greeley may have said, "Go West, young man," but Goran's mantra was just the opposite: "Go East, young doctors, but not too far."

Goran thus got involved in a chain of clinics called Centros de Esteticos, which were owned by an entrepreneur from Bel Air. I learned about this because Goran and I used to give second opinions to each other's patients (these visits were covered under all medical plans when surgery was recommended). At first, his patients were the standard middle class lot, but at some point, they were replaced by a lot of poor Latinos, many farm or factory workers whose big corporate employers did provide excellent health insurance, if little else, for them. Almost none of them needed the surgeries that Goran prescribed, and he became furious when I told them so. He blew up at me for trying to ruin his new business and stopped sending second opinions to me, though he slyly tried to co-opt me into the system by telling me about the fortune I could make by joining his practice. He invited me to come in with him to the Centros practice, to build my own patient list.

Karen, who spoke fluent Spanish and had both a good heart and a liberal spirit about aiding the less fortunate, encouraged me to break the Beverly Hills mold and "get real," as she had done as a schoolteacher. So I drove the Mercedes onto the 10 Freeway heading east, to three different Centros: downtown, El Monte, and the City of Commerce.

I would make this circuit, spending a few hours in each once a week, for three months, and saw nothing but sore throats, colds, and wax. No one needed plastic surgery. I did one broken nose repair in all the time I was there, then gave up and went back to Beverly Hills. How, I wondered, was Goran finding all these rhinoplasty patients? The answer was that he was making them up. I met a disgruntled anesthesiologist who told me how bad Goran was. Not only did his patients not need the procedures Goran was prescribing, but Goran wasn't even doing them. He was charging for them, to be sure. He would bill for a complex intranasal surgery that might take two hours, have the anesthesiologist put the patient under, come in and make a small cut in the patient's nose, which took all of five minutes, then go to an adjacent operating room and do the same thing. The patient would awake, all bandaged up, and since there had been nothing wrong with him to begin with, when the dressings were taken out of his nose a week later, he naturally felt better. Any nagging doubts were conquered by Goran's remarkable powers of salesmanship.

I was genuinely shocked and appalled, as was Karen. We thought about going to the authorities, but we didn't want to blow the whistle on a colleague. For one doctor to rat out another was considered the unkindest cut of all. Also, we knew that Goran was litigious. He had a team of lawyers, and he had already sued other doctors for defamation in some business deals that had gone wrong. He used the law like a club, to beat any enemies into submission. Goran's greed was so blatant, we figured someone else was bound to expose him sooner or later. But it never happened, and Goran got richer and richer, making fifty thousand or more a week on fake surgeries in the '80s, buying yachts and private jets and international vacation homes, all on the noses of these poor farm workers. Where was Cesar Chavez when we needed him?

The scary part was that Goran wasn't just one bad egg in a good basket. Some plastic surgeons would mine the Latino market, others the Asian, depending on what languages they had mastered. I spoke about it to a young Thai plastic surgeon who used to work with Goran, but he turned out to be doing the same thing with the wave of Thai immigrants who worked hard and had lots of disposable income, not to mention good insurance. Why, I asked him, would you do fake billing? His answer was a matter of professional survival. "You do it to build a practice. Once you're set up, then you can devote yourself to real patients and do good for them."

If you were rich to begin with, you didn't have to stoop so low to get started. There was a recently arrived Indian plastic surgeon who I worried would prey on the growing Indian community in suburban Cerritos. But he set himself up on Bedford Drive in Beverly Hills, where he succeeded mightily, and quickly. He came from a family of diamond kings in Coimbatore, near Madras. He bought a Bentley convertible, dated starlets, and rarely treated Indian patients unless they were friends of his powerful family. Word got out that he was an Indian prince, and Beverly Hills, obsessed with royalty, beat a path to his office.

Some doctors were simply too pretentious to deal with poor people, no matter how much money could be made, straight or crooked. There was a plastic surgeon who came from Queens who would show up in his office in polo whites, carrying his mallet, straight from the playing fields of Will Rogers Park in Pacific Palisades. He had taken the sport up when he went down to Brazil to learn a new buttocks-lifting procedure. Polo went to his head. He bribed emergency room nurses at the hospitals where he was on staff to let him know which patients had insurance. If they didn't, he'd avoid them by having the nurses call someone else, like me. Among the insured patients, he'd cherry-pick the best cases. The result was that he'd get to fix the broken nose while I was woken up at 3 a.m. for a nosebleed. Whenever I'd see him in the ER, I'd look to see if his polo pony was tethered at the entrance.

With such venal, self-absorbed, often bizarre doctors in my midst, it should come as no surprise that meeting Dexter Farnham restored my faith in my chosen profession and chosen locale. It was 1988, and we were at the doctors' lockers at Midway Hospital after finishing our surgeries. I had heard of him, and recognized his photos from medical society journals. He was always winning awards, inventing something new or lecturing in Ulan Bator or some impossibly far-flung locale. I knew he was the first plastic surgeon to have created teaching films for residents in training as well as for practicing doctors. I had seen his name on countless articles in many fields, not just plastic surgery, and he had devised innovative approaches to all sorts of surgical problems. If modern medicine had a Renaissance man, it was Dexter.

Not only was he a surgical Goliath, his tall and intimidating physicality matched his professional standing. I wanted to meet him, and, slipping out of my surgeon's greens, I put out my hand. Nearly as quickly, I dropped the name of Leslie Bernstein, my U.C. Davis mentor, which was always an "open sesame" among doctors of distinction, and it worked. The laconic, Olympian cowboy came down to earth, gave me the strongest handshake I had ever endured, and made me feel that I was the greatest young doctor on the planet. Because Dexter was so reserved and grand, any enthusiasm emanating from the man came across as the highest honor.

We talked about Leslie, about my work, about Dexter's latest innovations, and after half an hour, I felt so much at home with the man that I tried to get Treva, who was sick of doing all of Harold Brooks' breast implants for no credit and little money, a job as one of Dexter's scrub nurses. Dexter told me to have her call him. That night I stopped at the UCLA Medical School library to look Dexter up. What I found was one of the most impressive medical resumes I had ever seen. I was snowed. But when I called Treva to give her the good news that she might soon be working with this Socrates of surgery, she refused to even consider it. "He's a bastard and a slave driver", she said. Apparently, Dexter had fired a male nurse who was one of Treva's best friends, and solidarity in friendship meant more to her than career advancement. "Stay away from him," she warned. "He'll use you up and spit you out. He's the iceman."

"If only," I thought to myself. Dexter may have been a difficult boss to work for, I thought, but his brilliance and impressive bio and awards more than overshadowed her questionable diatribe. So when I met Dexter again, several years later, and he invited me to come work with him at his new office in East Los Angeles, I couldn't have been more honored. I had run into him several times at Cedars-Sinai when he stopped in to see if he could observe my surgeries. I was flattered that he was interested, nervous that he was there, but I couldn't say no. After watching me a few times, he told me that I was one of the best rhinoplasty surgeons he had ever seen, but that I needed to have more confidence in myself.

Now I could see the method in his madness of dropping by. Like so many surgeons, Dexter had decided to expand his practice. But he wasn't going to be another Goran Porec. He was pure class. Obviously the Hispanic market was the big one, but he was going in the front door, not the garbage chute, and he wanted me to be on his first team. Karen was thrilled when I told her. She was a Hispanophile, and had always wanted me to expand eastward, and here was a golden opportunity. I'd keep my Beverly Hills practice, and even burnish it by association with Dexter, who treated as many stars as anyone.

I thus began going once a week to Dexter's gleaming new clinic on Atlantic Boulevard in Monterey Park, which was a little Hong Kong as well as a little Mexico City, testament to Los Angeles' unmatched mix of cultures. Karen always said she preferred Mexicans to movie stars any day, perhaps because her mother worked for Jack Warner, to whom stars were just one big pain in the neck. Anyway I felt more noble helping the poor, and even more so at the side of Dexter Farnham, the father figure I had always been looking for in medicine, if not in life. He taught me all the newest procedures, including some on body parts below the neck, which had always been a boundary below which I wouldn't go. I did my first liposuction under Dexter's tutelage. He insisted that I learn how to do it, because lipo was rivaling noses and breasts as the most demanded procedure. I learned it so well that I even did some on several of Karen's relatives, who were thrilled to become Hollywood svelte.

Dexter challenged me, as I had never been challenged before, to be the best surgeon in a town overrun with them. He urged me to do things on my own terms, not their get-richer-quicker subterfuges. That the FBI could be beating down my door, impugning my integrity and that of the mentor who defined the term, was understandably a shock to my cancer-weakened system.

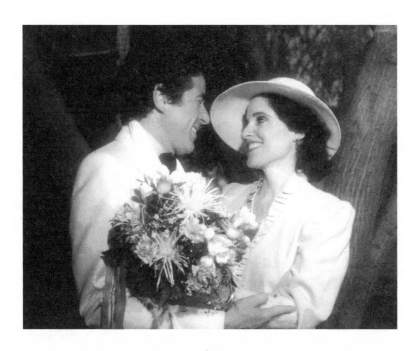

Love and Marriage

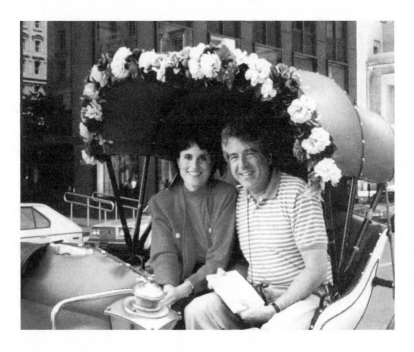

Chapter Five

THE BIG C

Despite being a sickly little kid, I was an amazingly healthy adult. Maybe all those childhood visits to the Medical Arts Building on the Bronx Concourse had conferred some magical immunity on me. Or maybe all that weightlifting and track in the Bronx had turned me around and saved me from being a disease-prone ninety-seven-pound weakling. Or maybe my number just hadn't come up. But it did. And how!

It was the summer of 1993. I was forty-eight years old. I was just emerging from a vicarious run of cancer with Karen's family that had started in 1989, when her father, Bob, died of pancreatic cancer. In 1992, her mother, Mimi, and sister, Gail, both got breast cancer and mastectomies within a year of each other. In that same year, 1992, my own dear mother finally succumbed to Parkinson's as well. I missed my mother terribly, but she had not been functional since her coma after my father's death of stomach cancer. I had gotten used to missing her spirit; now, with her body gone, the terrible finality had set in.

Still, I tried to look on the bright side. Mimi and Gail had survived. They were cancer-free and seemed to be doing well. My practice was a huge success. Karen and I had bought a wonderful new house in Bel Air, with Chinese rooms, Indian colonial rooms, English manor rooms, and 1940s film noir rooms, and we adored being there. We had also proudly created what we thought was one of the finest and most elaborate gardens LA had to offer.

The *LA Times* lauded us, and the garden was featured in several other publications. Our grounds were described as being the most lush and magnificent anywhere outside of the grand Huntington Gardens in San Marino. And we had spectacular ocean views, which the landlocked Huntington lacked. Karen's attention to detail and nurture had paid off: we had fragrant jasmine, agapanthus, lilies of the Nile, English foxgloves, hydrangeas, azaleas, roses, pansies, dahlias, and bleeding hearts. Karen had it timed so we had vibrant displays of color and heady perfumed scents all year round. This was a garden Monet would have loved to paint. In addition to our family of plants, we also had a wonderful family of four admirable cats: Dexter, Tinker, Doodle, and Wojge (a variant of old Norse), which may not have been exactly the family of kids we did not have, but we couldn't have loved anyone much more. I was spending a lot of time in the garden that summer, so I didn't give a second thought to the sunburn I had. But then the clouds finally rolled in and the redness failed to subside. One of Karen's friends noticed what she called a rash and said that I should have it checked out. Hey, I was the doctor, the head and neck plastic surgeon, the face man. What did she know? But after several months went by, the rash grew deeper and darker, and the skin began to feel increasingly sensitive. I finally made an appointment with my friend Marshall Rubin, a dermatologist who had offices in an adjacent building on Roxbury's doctors' row. I didn't want to waste a lot of time driving to Cedars or UCLA over what I was sure was nothing. I really saw Marshall to appease Karen, whose friend kept getting after her about how my rash hadn't healed and that a skin lesion that doesn't heal within two weeks could be cancer and must be investigated. This was one of the American Cancer Society's universally promulgated warning signs that doctors, used to a lifetime of false alarms, pay no attention to.

Perhaps I was in some sort of denial. But Karen warned me that, aside from my well-being, my red face could start scaring patients away. So I began to think about it, and my self-diagnosis was that it was rosacea, a benign kind of middle-aged acne that can be managed with steroid creams. It was no big deal, and Marshall would confirm this, and I could lay this one to rest. By the time I got to his office, the rash had begun to spread downward, from its initial beachhead to my face and neck.

Marshall took a look at me and said, Oh, it's just nerves. The lazy man's diagnosis. I was under less stress than usual, not more. If stress were the culprit, every doctor would have a very red face. Marshall then called in his three partners, all of whom were baffled. They stood there in their white coats, fists under their chins, nodding their heads. They each started mumbling possibilities: rosacea, vitamin deficiencies, lichen planus, pityriasis rosea, lupus. No one mentioned the C word, cancer. No one thought it was anything serious, just mysterious, given my otherwise excellent general health. But they agreed that the obvious thing to do was to settle the matter once and for all by doing a biopsy.

Marshall injected a small spot on my red forehead with xyolocaine, a numbing agent, and took a punch biopsy with a cylindrical instrument that looks like a hole puncher. The specimen, a tiny sliver of skin, was then sent to a pathology laboratory for analysis. I was completely detached from the procedure. It was my skin, but once it had been removed, it wasn't me anymore. I had a terrible time confronting the reality of illness. I could not contemplate the idea of my dying. This biopsy challenged my complacency and cast my mortality into the glaring reality of my own measurable existence. And yet I remained in denial. Physicians often forget that it is only a matter of time before we are all patients, with vulnerability and feelings of isolation. Still, being a physician, I rationalized ways to protect myself. Not me, I thought. No way. My rash and symptoms could be representative of a hundred less serious diseases than cancer.

While we waited for the pathology report, Karen, who was an extreme hypochondriac, decided I had caught leprosy from one of Dexter's exotic patients in his East LA office. She began thinking of the jungles of Central America, and poisonous plants and giant insects, and before long, she was convinced she was married to the Elephant Man, at least in the making. For someone with such an overheated imagination, Karen proved to be incredibly strong with the reality of her family's cancers. She had no hospitalphobia; she was there for all of them, and never lost her composure. It was just when it came to herself, and now me, that she would freak out, something she attributed to seeing her beloved grandmother die a grisly death of breast cancer when Karen was just a little girl.

Karen's overreaction was her own defense mechanism against bad news. When the final diagnosis came in that her brain tumor was a headache or her stomach cancer was heartburn, she embraced the relief she felt and lived her life that much more fully. So she was overreacting on my behalf, preparing for the worst, as so many Jews, to whom the worst has happened over the centuries, tend to do, but secretly expecting the best. If she prepared for leprosy, all she was really anticipating was eczema. But no classical Jew could dare articulate optimism. That would be hubris, or, in Yiddish, *kinahurra*, which meant that the evil eye would look ill upon those who spoke too well of themselves.

And that was all it was, when the biopsy came back. I returned to Marshall's office, where he gave me the good news. All the biopsy showed was "nonspecific inflammation." He would have sent me home at that point with some sample salves, but I wanted to be more specific than he did. Having put on my Sherlock Holmes hat, I had decided that what I might have was lupus, the telltale clue being that the rash started following my exposure to sunlight. Lupus was a connective tissue disease of unknown origin that was most prevalent in women between the ages of fifteen and thirty-five. The main symptoms are awful joint pain, fever, coughing, and pericarditis, or inflammation of the heart lining. I had none of the above, but the sun-prompted rash was a major unique symptom, although rarely the first one. Yet I knew anything was possible, and I wanted to go further. Lupus could be fatal if not treated.

Marshall couldn't have cared less. He and his colleagues were focused on a new line of beauty and anti-aging products they had just created; their offices were being used to film advertising spots and infomercials. That's where the money was, in their minds: in snake oil, not in curing actual diseases. I thanked Marshall and went to my office to call a rheumatologist friend named Kevin Porter. Rheumatology was the field lupus would fall under, and Kevin was a leader in it. But I didn't tell Karen, not yet. Instead I made a joke out of her concern. "You're not getting that holiday in Molokai," I said, referring to the Hawaiian isle that had once been the world's most famous leper colony. "EGBOK." EGBOK was an acronym we had picked up from a local radio talk show: Everything's Gonna Be O.K. Without being hubristic and summoning the evil eye, we used to reassure each other with it before we went to sleep. It was our own little verbal talisman, and it had served us well. EGBOK.

I had several appointments with Kevin, a no-nonsense doctor whom I had first worked with twenty years before. I had taken on a female patient with a hole in her nose and a collapsed bridge. Other doctors had shunned her, believing that the nasal collapse was caused by a cocaine addiction. The other doctors assumed she was simply trying to get a nose job covered by her insurance, which, as a rule, did not like to "enable" drug addicts. I didn't see her as an addict at all, but as a woman with a problem, which I, proud of myself as a smart diagnostician, believed to be a joint disorder called relapsing polychondritis, which attacked cartilage. So I sent her to Kevin the joint man, who decided I was a genius, and we stayed in touch. When this poor woman died of her condition a decade later, Kevin called me up in tears. Most doctors don't show any emotion at all.

Kevin did a battery of esoteric blood tests, X-rays, EKGs and the like to rule lupus out—or in. Everything was negative, except for one single lab assay, which was borderline positive. Kevin, a good internist as well as a specialist, wasn't at all convinced I had lupus, but my rash had by now spread onto my shoulders and chest. Also, my scalp was becoming extra sensitive. It was hard to comb or brush my hair, and soon hurt to shampoo. My face remained suspiciously red. I worried that my patients would think I had become a florid alcoholic, though I didn't want to start apologizing for it or blaming it on too much gardening, for fear of calling attention to something they might not even have noticed. Never complain, never explain, was the old saying. I refused to wear makeup, which I called fakeup. Still, I had grotesque visions of becoming that Elephant Man with pachydermia, as it was known. Maybe that trip to Molokai had been canceled too soon.

Months had gone by with no improvement, and I couldn't keep Karen in the dark when she could see the rash so clearly. She did keep her cool, and not only shampooed my hair with her gentle touch, but experimented with vitamin creams and every beauty lotion she had in her formidable arsenal, which sometimes resembled the perfume-fragrant ground floor of Saks Fifth Avenue. She remained calm, as did I. It was just a rash. I was strong as a horse, doing as many as three surgeries a day. I felt terrific, except for my scalp. I had been to two big-time doctors, or at least one doctor and one cosmetician. Neither was worried. Why should we be?

But Kevin wouldn't rest. He suggested I go to a more serious dermatologist, out of Beverly Hills, in the less fashionable Wilshire Boulevard area known as the Miracle Mile. The area may have been a miracle in the Roaring Twenties, but now it was a miracle if you didn't get mugged when you walked the desolate stretch after dark. Still, the doctor there, Leonard Williams, insisted on doing another punch biopsy, this time of my upper chest, so there would be no scarring. I returned to his office a week later to get the results. By this point, all these doctors' visits were beginning to feel like a waste of time. I hadn't been a patient since I was a teenager, and medicine, at least what I could see, hadn't come very far in three decades. Today was going to be my last day as a patient. I would just learn to live with whatever bizarre thing this was, and one day it would probably just go away. When the nurse led me into Williams' spartan office, I had to wait a long time. Bored, I looked all around. On his desk I could see, upside down, my name on a sheet of paper. This was my biopsy report. But then my heart sank. The sheet of paper was filled and stapled to other pages. Negative reports showed a lot of white space. The words "normal" or "within normal limits" or "nonspecific inflammation" don't take that much room. My stomach sank, as if my plane had hit a bad air pocket. Darkness enveloped me. I hadn't felt fear before, and now, before I could get up and read the awful truth, the sheer volume of this truth made me jump to the worst possible conclusion. I couldn't believe a sheath of papers could make a man, a surgeon, tremble, but I was shaking like a leaf.

Just as I was getting up to read the bad news, Williams came in and saved me the trouble. "You have cancer," he said, dispensing with any preamble. I wasn't sure what he was going to say. I almost thought he was going to say, "You have lupus," which would have been bad enough, a story of pain and diminishing returns until…But cancer was worse, far worse, the worst word in my dictionary.

Although I was destroyed by the message, I respected his austere directness. Ashes to ashes. I had had to give bad news before, and nothing was harder. It was an awesome burden to impart to another human being, that this thing called life, with all its joys and sorrows, pleasures and pains, was coming to an ignominious end, as all ends necessarily must be, regardless of the glories that may have gone before. Nothingness was ignominious, any way you cut it. For all the deaths I had observed, this was the first time I understood, deep in my viscera, that life, wonderful life, did not go on forever. Now my only question was the matter of time. How much, and how bad?

I let the doctor do all the talking. I was speechless. He told me how he had ordered DNA studies, and that I had blood cancer. Further testing would have to be done to determine whether it was lymphoma, leukemia, or multiple myeloma. None of it was good, but Williams was betting that it was lymphoma, the best of a fatal lot. But he was just a dermatologist, and he was going to send me back to Kevin Porter to organize the procedure that would lead to the final diagnosis. Every word he used like "final," whatever the context, had the ring of a death knell.

My mind raced back thirty years to med school and everything I knew about lymphoma, which was cancer of the lymph system, which produces the lymphocytes, one of the white blood cells that is the key weapon of the body's immune system. Cancer cells manage to trick their way past the Trojan wall of the lymph system, which somehow doesn't recognize them as foreign. They begin growing out of control, causing the lymph glands to get bigger and bigger, and, well, you can imagine the rest. I had thus been fooled by the Trojan horse of cancer. How could my damn body have been so trusting, so naïve, so stupid?

To allow me a glimmer of hope, and as a doctor I knew it was the stuff of fireflies not beacons, Williams did allow that the whole process might, and he emphasized might, be benign. It was highly unusual for an initial cancer diagnosis like this to be made from a skin sample. Maybe the pathology lab was wrong. Maybe, maybe, maybe… Miracles did happen, but I wasn't counting on them. I staggered out into the bright Los Angeles afternoon sunshine, the sunshine of hope and dreams. I was in a daze. It was as if I had been mugged, stabbed, left for dead. The darkest alleys of the South Bronx would have seemed more inviting than this once glorious stretch of Wilshire Boulevard, the boulevard of dreams, the Miracle Mile. Now the dreams were shattered, lying in pieces in the hellish sun. All I could think of was the Rolling Stones' "Paint It Black."

I suddenly realized that although my life might be over, my day was not. I had an office full of patients with appointments that I had to see. My first instinct was to cancel, but, then again, my first instinct was to cancel the rest of my life. Did my Hippocratic oath compel me to "bop till I dropped," to keep treating patients until I was too sick to don the white coat? As a plastic surgeon, most of my patients had brief windows of exposure to me. I'd do the surgery, and they would hopefully be happy and go on with their lives. Yes, there were the plastic surgery junkies who'd go from nose job to facelift to lipo, to implants, but I avoided those types. I could retire, go off to die in peace, and nobody would miss me. Those were the dark thoughts that filled my mind on the Miracle Mile. A cancer diagnosis can do that, even to the toughest of us. Then I pulled it all together, got in the Mercedes, and drove back to work. EGBOK. I was a pro. I was a winner. Winners never quit.

The hardest part was figuring out how to break the news to Karen. I thought about lying, but Karen was a human polygraph. She had mendacity ESP. You couldn't fool her. The minute I walked into the office and gave a big hearty smile to all my waiting patients, Karen spotted the bluff. "It's bad, isn't it?" she said, cornering me in my office. So I told her, tempering the blow by reminding her how normal all my blood and other tests were, and raising the specter of a possible misreading or false alarm. Instead of breaking down, Karen just gazed at me with her huge, dazzling green eyes—"them there eyes" as the Billie Holiday song went that I always thought of as Karen's song ("They make me feel happy. They make me feel blue. No stallin'. I'm fallin'. Going in a big way for sweet little you…")—and X-rayed me with all her love and compassion. Then she drew close to me and took my hand. And then she held me to herself and kissed me. She was incredibly strong, far stronger than I was, and her strength gave me strength, the strength to beat this damn thing, whatever it was. We didn't say a word, not even EGBOK. I just drank in the power of her eyes, the healing power, the power of love. I straightened up my desk and got ready for my first patient.

Kevin Porter sent me to his "cancer guy," Herb Bloomfield, who, like Kevin, had a suite in the Cedars-Sinai Office Towers. After the doctors' rows of Bedford and Roxbury, the Towers was the most likely place in Los Angeles to spot movie stars, who happened to get sick like ordinary mortals. And now like me. Herb was the most nondescript doctor I could imagine. He had as little personality as he had physical distinction. But Kevin said he was brilliant, and I trusted Kevin. Trust is how you pick doctors. There is no Zagat. It's a most imperfect science, choosing doctors, and I assumed that since I was in the club, my choices would be the most informed possible. I could look up degrees and credentials, but what it came down to in the end was this chain letter of trust, from one doctor to another and on to the patient. Now I was in the chain.

With Herb I wasn't looking for Mr. Congeniality; I was looking for a diagnosis. After a long and, to me, repetitious examining process, I called his attention to a tiny sub-pea-sized swelling in my neck just below my earlobe. I had noticed it throughout the whole year I had had this rash, but I had written it off as a reaction to my low-grade scalp irritation, or infection, or whatever it was. That's what lymph glands do; they swell up to fight infection. No other doctor had paid any attention to it, and neither had I, a head and neck surgeon who was constantly palpating my patients' lymph nodes to see if those inflamed tonsils or infected sinuses had produced a lymphatic reaction. "Swollen glands" was a common phenomenon, and here I had a gland that was slightly, almost imperceptibly enlarged, which I had basically ignored as nothing when I thought I had nothing. But now I had something, and the ominous look on Herb's face when he felt the pea in my neck spelled big trouble in River City.

Herb wanted me to get the lump biopsied, which was a minor operation. He also wanted me to get a bone marrow biopsy, which was a major pain. First, the lump. I went to another good surgeon at Cedars whom I knew, Dr. Wolf Blaufels, who didn't believe the lump was "clinically important," which meant having some effect or role in the disease process, but I pressed him to excise it and examine it. This involved real surgery, surgery I had done, and I knew exactly what the risks were when you cut someone's neck, which is what had to be done to me to get the gland. There were distinct possibilities of bleeding, infection, swelling, injury to nerves that could affect speech and swallowing. Talk about the shoe on the other foot. I remembered the William Hurt film *The Doctor*, in which an arrogant cardiac surgeon is humbled, and beyond, when he gets throat cancer. What new empathy I felt for the poor visitors to my office.

Karen did come with me to Cedars for this surgery. My predicament really hit me when I changed for the OR, not into my green scrub suit, where I was the boss, but into a patient gown. Being wheeled on a stretcher into the OR, looking straight up, gave me a new perspective, in more ways than one. I thought I knew this particular OR in every way, for I had worked here many times. But on the flat side of the gurney, I found I didn't know it at all. How much better, I thought, to give rather than to receive. The next thing I remembered was waking up in the recovery room, a big bandage on my neck. All had gone perfectly, and there were no ill effects, other than the endless days' wait for the pathology report.

Next, Herb, the cancer man, did the bone marrow biopsy. This involved jamming a horse-sized needle into my hip bone to take a sample of my marrow. As I was being read the consent form, with its litany of terrifying risks, I realized that no matter how beautiful I thought I was going to make my patients, I was still inflicting major bodily injury on them, way beyond conventional assault and battery. Healthy patients were turned into sick patients. In my case, beauty had nothing to do with it. This was a matter of life and death, so whatever the horror, it was life and had to be endured. The needle looked like a railroad spike, an ominous piece of stainless steel.

Herb numbed only my skin, no deeper, promising me it wasn't going to hurt. What a lie! Maybe he was of the opinion that doctors feel no pain. The aspiration needle was inserted and, with extreme force, was pushed through the outer shell, or cortex, of the bone. I heard a crack and felt the penetration, which made me totally nauseated and awash with anxiety. There was my mortality, stabbing me in the back, soon after it had slit my throat. There was nothing my caduceus shield or MD degree could protect me from. I heard a sucking sound, which was the marrow being taken out of me, the marrow, the chief source of red blood cell production, the mythical source of animal vigor in health, the delicacy in osso buco, the Italian veal shank dish. I now understood the expression "chilled down to the marrow."

Once they got the marrow, I was sent for a CAT scan of my body cavities to see if any other lymph glands, or anything else, had grown to an abnormal size. The intense claustrophobia of being stuck motionless in a dark cocoon lasted over an hour, but this was the final event of the investigation. I was told I would be called to schedule a follow-up appointment when all the results were in and could be analyzed. That call came sooner rather than later, while I was at home feeding the cats. It was Herb himself. He said he knew I wanted to know. Because he lacked any charm whatsoever, and had no bedside manner, I think he preferred the phone, as it minimized the human factor for him.

"You have non-Hodgkins lymphoma," he said flatly, an emotionless version of those canned calls that tell you you've won a free trip to a Carson City timeshare. He didn't really elaborate beyond defining the categories of the disease that had been diagnosed. "Call my office tomorrow to set up an appointment." No "I'm sorry," no "We're gonna beat this sucker" pep talk. No nothing. Just the facts, ma'am, just the facts.

My initial reaction was a strange relief. It was brutal news, but it was better than multiple myeloma, which was basically death after two years of hell, or most leukemias, which were basically death a lot quicker, but less grisly. From what I could remember, I might get four or five years with NHL. Of course I wanted a life, my life, a long life. I wasn't even fifty. But four or five years were better than the other possibilities, way better. It's amazing how your mind can adjust to adversity. Then I remembered that Jackie Onassis had recently died of NHL at 64, and very quickly. If the most fabulous, most connected woman on earth couldn't lick the Big C, what hope was there for mere mortals, even a surgeon like me? I didn't want to go gently into that good night. I wanted to live. Why me? I thought, like every other poor sucker who gets hit in the gut with the bad news. Why me?

"It's only non-Hodgkins lymphoma," I quickly told Karen, who had been by my side for the operations at Cedars. Her normally sparkling eyes became sad and sympathetic, not fearful, almost as if she had expected the bad news. Then gentle tears started to flow. The cancer curse was striking into the heart of her life once again. How much cancer could one family take? She hugged me and tried to be as strong as she could. I tried to be even stronger, assuring her

I would fight and beat this thing, that lots of people lived long, full lives with NHL.

I had known for at least the last fifteen years that I could not lie to Karen, even if I wanted to. Either I was a bad liar or she had an extraordinary sense of perception. She was rarely fooled by anyone. At times it seemed uncanny. Of course, now I was shooting from the hip, not having read about the disease for thirty years. What I was really thinking about were the celebs I had read about who had quick downhhill progressions: Jackie O and Senator Paul Tsongas, to name two recent victims. But this was one time Karen didn't read my mind. Or maybe she did and didn't want to tell me.

That was one sad night in Bel Air. Once Karen had fallen asleep, I stole down to my medical library to read all about my new nemesis: NHL. It was not fun reading. There were countless pages of medical minutiae. The disease was extremely complicated, with many subdivisions. Herb had told me in our charming call that I had a version called indolent, follicular, small B-cell NHL. I was grateful I didn't have the pirhana, or psychotic, or supercharged versions, which were my shorthand for the more aggressive subtypes. The worst part was reading the mortality tables, which hadn't changed much from when I was in med school. There was a 50–60 percent death rate within the first six to eight years. There it was in black and white, but at least I wasn't going to be dead in months, like in pancreatic or esophageal cancer, or in some of the more vicious leukemias. I took a lot of courage from that. I knew medicine was moving very fast, and in the few years I had ahead of me, lots of good things might happen. Or at least, that's what I kept telling myself, to help me fall asleep.

The next day, Herb Bloomfield was his usual barrel of laughs. He told me I was in Stage IV of the disease, meaning that it had spread all over my body. What was Stage V, I asked him. He replied that there was no Stage V. When I pressed him about what we were going to do, his answer was "watch and wait." That meant we would do nothing, watching for the disease to progress, get aggressive, and cause pain and suffering, which it wasn't now. Once it did that, then I would start a course of chemotherapy that would, if it worked, send it into remission, for how long no one could know. The cancer man stressed that I had an incurable disease. Remission and cure are two different things. Remission is simply a time out. Herb urged me not to read the literature on NHL. I told him that it was too late. I left glad for the moment that I was able to beg the question of chemotherapy, which is a toxic adventure at best, and at worst a hell on earth that makes you wonder whether chasing a dwindling life is worth all the horror and suffering.

Karen and I decided we would not tell anyone, not even her family, about my illness. Nobody wants to be treated, much less operated on, by a dying doctor. But we were still worried about my red face. Because of the short-term nature of my practice, I could use the sunburn excuse for most patients, who would be out of the office in the time it took such a burn to wear off. I would be the perpetual boy of summer. It was an excuse that would play only in Southern California, though I worried how long I would actually need to make it. Any day, the indolence of my NHL could mutate into attack, and that would be the end of my career, not to mention my life.

The only other person I told my secret to was Dexter. Since I worked so closely with him, I felt it my professional responsibility to make a full disclosure. I thought he'd tell me to quit, but instead he exhorted me to keep working, and working even harder. "It's the work that makes you feel as good as you do. You've got a gift, Alvin. Don't squander it on self-pity. You're a genius with your hands. You owe it to our patients. You're a healer, a creator, a maker. You're not an invalid. Hell, do you feel sick? You're only as sick as you feel. Fuck the biopsies."

I appreciated the pep talk and show of confidence, but Dexter was more than a revival preacher. He truly believed the twelve-step gospel, and he applied it to any illness, not merely drug addiction or alcoholism. One day at a time was his credo, and he got me thinking the same way. I owed my mental health in this awful crisis to his positive approach, and to his drill sergeant's rigor about making me work night and day. Even though at the time I got sick no more than 10 percent of my practice came from Dexter's East LA clinic, in 1995 he opened the Beverwil Surgery Center, and he fed me all the work I could handle. "Don't waste your energies chasing business. I've got all the business there is. And don't waste your precious time on billings and paperwork. I'll do it all for you. You just use your gift. You just operate. I'll take care of the rest."

The idea of freeing myself from a growing mountain of bureaucratic red tape was an offer I could not refuse. When you've got a terminal illness, that red tape seems even more meaningless than it normally does. While I continued to run my own Beverly Hills office practice, I now turned over Dexter's East LA clinic patient billing and paperwork to him. A big load was lifted. Cancer changes your priorities. You focus on what you love; you eliminate what you hate. I recalled the old Guy Lombardo standard from the 1940s, a staple of New Year's celebrations: "Enjoy yourself, it's later than you think. Enjoy yourself, while you're still in the pink." I was pink, to be sure, and Dexter's heartfelt advice to follow my bliss seemed just what the doctor ordered.

A year of lymphoma indolence and career industry went by. I still felt fine. I was doing dozens of surgeries a month. I loved my life, even with the sword of Damocles perched millimeters from my red neck. In 1996, Karen and I went to Washington DC for a meeting of the Facial Plastic Surgery Society. The top surgeons from all over the country were there, each paying obeisance when I mentioned that I worked with Dexter Farnham. I felt great about myself, except when I looked in the mirror and saw my florid face and thinning hair. One of my strongest features was my preternaturally thick Samsonian locks. But now my scalp was not only aching; it was thinning. Oh, sweet bird of youth. My boyish looks were finally going, and I hated the idea of being bald almost, a distant almost, as much as I hated dying. Death was still abstract. Hair loss was concrete.

A trade fair of dermatological products accompanied the conference. At the time, the carbon dioxide laser skin tightening and wrinkle removing procedure was coming into vogue, and one of its side effects was a red face that lasted for months. A huge number of cosmetics were entering the market to camouflage this redness, and Karen bought one of each to try out. Back at the hotel, she tried one makeup on me after another. Finally she found one that looked the least fake, a liquid that didn't cake, and she insisted I use it. The only real drawback, aside from turning me into a drag queen, was that it would bleed all over my shirt collars. I quickly became skillful at keeping it mostly on my face and blending it into the top of my neck. If my career in plastic surgery ever failed, and I was alive, I knew I had a second chance as a makeup artist.

I was praying for as much time as I could have. The conference had made me excited about being a plastic surgeon at the dawn of a golden age of this practice. New developments were coming every day: lasers, computer imaging, all kinds of high-tech procedures, revolutionary skin products, new approaches to liposuction, facial implants, forehead lifts, and on and on. A paradigm shift was taking place. Dexter was a leader in it, and I was right by his side. I was in the right place at the right time. All I wanted was to stay there.

After the conference, Karen and I rented a car to drive down the Shenandoah Parkway to Charlottesville at the peak of fall foliage, of which we are deprived in Southern California; we made the trip to visit her niece, an archaeology graduate student at the University of Virginia. Charlottesville is probably the most beautiful university town outside of Oxford and Cambridge, and I felt a special awe visiting Monticello and walking in the giant footsteps of our most scientific president, Thomas Jefferson.

I also felt something else: a lump in my groin. I was strolling alone on a hill near Monticello surveying God's country and suddenly I stopped short, in a cold sweat. What I first took to be a fold in my pants did not fall away as I shook my leg. With no one around, I put my hand inside my trousers and palpated the area. I felt not one, or two, but multiple small masses on both sides of my inner thigh. Then I felt the rest of my body, my armpits, my neck. Nothing. I didn't tell Karen, for fear of ruining our idyllic vacation, our year of hope. But the cancer had begun to spread. The age of indolence was over. The war was about to begin.

Chapter Six

DEAD MAN WALKING

My very first thought upon feeling those ominous lumps in my groin was a curiosity as to what Thomas Jefferson had died of. Even a doctor's subconscious may be programmed to react scientifically. It was better than panic or self-pity, which were definitely lurking in the wings. I could feel a repressed horror that my cancer was suddenly exploding, that my body was careening out of control. But I was able to table those thoughts. After all, I was luxuriating in one of the most serene spots on earth. If I hadn't noticed those damn lumps, I would have thought I was Superman, invincible. I doubted that Jefferson, a gardener and a man of science (sort of, with poetic license) like myself, would have panicked under similar circumstances, so neither would I. I let Dr. Reiter tell patient Reiter, "You have cancer. It's changed its course. It's getting aggressive. We'll treat it."

I remembered that, even in his malarial times, Jefferson lived until a ripe old age, riper than mine by three decades. They say life is unfair, but death is arrogantly fickle. Still, my cinematic role model for my own self-image as a doctor remained John Wayne as the pilot of the supposedly doomed plane in *The High and the Mighty*. As the Duke's earthborn medical counterpart, my mission had always been to use all my skills, my best instincts, and my compassion for my patients to beat whatever odds they were up against. But then again, I wasn't a cancer doctor, and I wasn't usually dealing with life and death situations, just helping people look better and feel better.

Now the reality was crashing in. John Wayne had been licked by the Big C. Jacqueline Kennedy Onassis, who I imagined had the best medical care money and fame could buy on earth, had gone down to the Big C, my Big C, in a matter of months. I had felt those lumps in others, and I could describe them by the book: firm, nodular, non-tender, non-mobile. But that was by the medical book, not the Book of the Dead, which is what it felt like when those lumps were your own. Those lumps could mean only one thing, that my "indolent" non-Hodgkin's lymphoma, had gotten off its lazy ass and was looking to kick mine, like an angry monster awakened from its torpor.

As a doctor, I knew what could be done, and I knew the odds were against me. Those odds on survival of longer than five years were quoted at less than fifty-fifty, but, being a precision man, I knew that actually there was a more than a 60 percent chance that I would be dead in less than three years, because I had already survived two years since the discovery of the cancer, and on the median, I had only three to go. Those were bad odds. I also knew the arsenal at my disposal against the monster NHL, and that arsenal, the dreaded and lethal chemotherapy, was likely to hurt me as much as it would hurt the monster. It was like when your parents were going to spank you, they would say, "This is going to hurt me more than you." Yes, I knew a lot. That knowledge could be power, yet it could also be a dangerous thing.

I was a big man, a wise man, a man of science, but only in the "good" 40 percent, the longer-term survival, where I could play for time and have a life. In the other sixty, the "bad" sixty, reason did me no good whatsoever. That bad sixty was the Great Unknown, the netherland of luck, chance, superstition, spirituality. That's where faith came in, and that was terra incognita for this medicine man, who lived by reason and science. If anything truly frightened me in the beautiful Jeffersonian hills, those hills of reason and science, it was the notion that at that moment, I was rolling the dice in the big casino of life and death, and I was anything but a betting man. I lived for control, and now I had lost it.

More movie images flashed in my head. I never had that much time for movies, even less for books, but now those indelible frames were crowding the multiplex of my rattled mind. There was Clint Eastwood in *Dirty Harry* asking the mugger, "Are you feeling lucky, punk?" just before he said his big line, "Go ahead, make my day." Well, I was one punk who wasn't feeling lucky. I had felt fortunate before. I had felt blessed often. But I had never felt "lucky." I had never been a gambler, but now I was being forced to play the odds—the deadly odds.

Despite my massive anxieties, the last thing I wanted to do at the moment was ruin Karen's vacation. Karen was the main reason I felt blessed, and she had had enough cancer in her family. To add me to the list of potential casualties was a cruel joke. My cancer was our Big Unmentionable, lying as dormant in our everyday lives as it had lain in my body. It wasn't as if it was the elephant in the room; aside from my rash, I had no other evidence of cancer, and I felt wonderful. Why dwell on dark matters when so much sunshine was beaming in? In any case, Karen and I couldn't have been having a happier time than on this magnificent Southern autumn, so I did my utmost to play it cool, knowing that Karen had the investigative instincts of Sherlock Holmes. Somehow I pulled it off for the next few days, hiking, antiquing, touring plantations, eating lots of Southern fried foods.

The lapse in my otherwise fairly austere dietary habits did pique Karen's curiosity. Why order steamed vegetables if you're going to be dead soon? Why not go out with a delicious cholesterol bang, with hush puppies, fried catfish, green beans stewed in lard, and pork skin "cracklins." Of course, what I said was that it was a shame to be in Virginia and remain on the Beverly Hills nonfat salad plan, but somehow Karen didn't buy it, and I restrained all future epicurean impulses. I also restrained all impulses to call Herb Bloomfield, even from the secrecy of a pay phone, to talk about my lumps. It was a true command performance. Soon, however, the idyll was over. Back in Los Angeles, I called Herb, Mr. Personality, and went over to his office during a lunch hour when Karen went shopping. Herb did a quick exam, made few comments on my findings other than agreeing, without any emotion, that yes, apparently the cancer had indeed spread, and ordered a new CAT scan. It was set up for a weekday afternoon, necessitating my leaving the office and thus breaking the grim tidings to Karen the morning of the appointment. As I had feared, she broke down sobbing. "I'm going to lose my husband to cancer," she despaired, cursing the demon disease that seemed to have it in for everyone she loved. But then she pulled herself together, reminding herself that her mother and sister were still very much alive, and so was I. She joked that she "knew" something was wrong when I ordered the glory that was grease. She gave me a big hug and an EGBOK and sent me across the street to the Rox-San Medical Building (named for its coordinates, Roxbury Drive and Santa Monica Boulevard), which contained a major imaging center.

The worst part was, and is, the waiting. I waited an hour for the radiologist, waited another hour for the results. Aside from the claustrophobia, the scan was a piece of cake, albeit one laced with arsenic. I started worrying about radiation, especially when the scan tech hid behind a shield. Then again, who was I kidding? I already had cancer. What the hell would I be hiding from?

Normally I would have had to wait a day or more to get the results from Herb. I somehow was able to convince the radiologist that as a doctor I could "handle" the bad tidings that I was sure of getting. I think this radiologist was so starved for human contact that he let his guard down to chat with me person to person. He put the films up on a view box in a dark room, and there I was, cancer-ridden, in black and white. I stared at those nodes, paraaortic nodes as they were called. It was weird looking at my body, the body that had betrayed me. I felt so good outside; I looked so bad inside. Here was my future, in shades of gray, and that future was as grim as its hue. Here it was: the awful truth. My cancer had gone ballistic; metastatic was the medical word. All doubts were erased, all my worst fears realized.

I walked back out into that endless have-a-nice-day cheery California sunshine and crossed the street to my office. Would the chemo allow me to keep things going? Nobody likes being treated by a dying doctor. It just doesn't inspire confidence. Cancer is like cooties. If I were able to keep working, I would have to keep this illness a dark secret, which might not be so easy to do once my weight started dropping and all my hair had fallen out.

But first I had to tell Karen. The long corridor leading to my office seemed like the last mile in a prison. I faked a big smile for my receptionist, then went to my private office, where Karen joined me. Despite an attempt to seem chipper, my long face betrayed me. Karen must have been hoping against hope, for she suddenly broke down behind the closed door. "Hey, I'll get treatment, that's all," I tried to assure her, as I called Herb to set up a follow-up appointment, fortunately for the next day. Somehow my medical training diminished my layman's terror of chemo, even though I was well aware of the awful side effects: the pain, the nausea, the almost inevitable baldness, the excruciatingly erosive mouth sores, the crushing fatigue, and more. But surgery hurt, too, and I did it every day. So I regarded it as getting a dose of my own medicine. I still could not conceive of my own death, not now. I had an office full of patients to take care of, a wife to love, cats to feed, plants to water. There was no time in my life for death.

The next day, Herb laid out the course of chemo. He offered no prognosis whatsoever, no sense of optimism, no sense of hope. It wasn't as if he were dwelling on the bad odds. He just wasn't a hopeful sort; maybe no oncologist was. It was a specialty of grim reapers. He did warn me, "Don't read the textbooks." Fat chance. I was looking for good news, not bad, information on new treatments that Herb, a major player in his field, surely knew about but didn't want to discuss.

I did read about the chemo drug Herb had chosen for me, Fludarabine, which would have terrified the Terminator. Although the usual side effects of nausea and hair loss were less likely, the bigger risk here was a much higher incidence of aplastic anemia, a blood disorder that rapidly kills you. However, of the other drugs Herb had been considering, one could cause irreversible heart damage, the other peripheral nerve damage. As a surgeon, I preferred to risk death rather than the loss of my hands, so I opted for the Fludarabine as the least of the three evils. My concern for my practice showed that I was basically optimistic that things would somehow work out, though it may not have seemed like it at the time.

Even scarier than the prospect of chemo was the "minor" operation I had to have to start the process: a plastic port would be installed under my clavicle into which the Fludarabine would be dripped for the first five days of every month. The Cedars vascular surgeon Herb sent me to, who had red hair and freckles and reminded me of Howdy Doody, was a garrulous talk show host by comparison to Herb. He may have also been a bit of a sadist, given the barely concealed glee he took in enumerating all that could go wrong with the procedure, including collapsed veins, hemorrhage, death. But if I didn't get the port, the frequency of the chemo would take a grueling toll on my veins. I had no choice but to sign the surgical consent, and we set a date a few weeks away to do the deed. Any port in a storm, I said to myself. Gallows humor was better than no humor at all.

Soon after all the bad news hit, Karen's mother, Mimi, gave a family "solidarity" dinner, for which she made her special roast chicken in my honor. Mimi, though she had looked a lot like Carole Lombard when she was young, always reminded me of the all-American Betty White on *The Golden Girls*. She was perky and chipper, the most positive person I knew. Mimi was a true trooper, surviving the loss of her beloved husband in 1988, surviving her own breast cancer even now. She was fortunate to have a wonderful new man in her life, proving love can conquer all, at any age. Her boyfriend, Dave, was a retired tycoon in his eighties who exploded the Beverly Hills stereotype that old tycoons were like Daddy Warbucks, surrounding themselves with Anna Nicole Smith type pneumatic gold diggers who had been reconstructed by my plastic surgery colleagues so that they could land the likes of Dave. But Dave was a solid citizen who wanted true love and companionship, not a trophy bimbo and a posthumous estate battle. Karen's sister, Gail, also a cancer survivor, was at the dinner, though her lawyer husband, Lee, was absent.

I guess I was a cancer survivor myself, according to the current definition, which states that anyone with a diagnosis of cancer is automatically a survivor. So everyone is a survivor until they die, with or without the cancer. I had always assumed that being a survivor meant that you had been cured. In any case, I hated the "C" word, preferring to refer to my condition as "my lymphoma." The word "lymph" sounded like "nymph," the semidivine maidens of Greek mythology who lived in the woods near lakes and rivers; it evoked images of clear liquids, of limpid pools. "He leadeth me beside the still waters, he restoreth my soul…" Lymphoma sounded to me like the name of a flower. That was the gardener in me. But now it was the fleur du mal, the flower of evil. Still, I preferred the "L" word to the "C" word, but oddly enough, nobody at the dinner ever mentioned either word. It was all unspoken, a silent show of support, yet it felt good to have family around me.

Even before I had my port surgery, Herb had started me on a drug called Leukeran, which was a variant of the poisonous nitrogen mustard gas that was used by the Germans against the Allies in World War I. The tablets were tiny, but within half an hour of taking my first one, I felt desperately ill, as if I had been gassed myself. I could barely move. A black cloud engulfed me. I stopped taking the pills immediately. Then I thought it might be psychosomatic. After all, this was the first time I had actually taken something for my cancer, or lymphoma, whatever the disease was going to be called, and perhaps I was reacting emotionally rather than physically. So the next day I started again and got just as sick. This time, though, I stuck with it, thinking the ill effects would wear off. They didn't, and after a month of debilitating malaise, I was a bad patient and stopped taking my medicine. I did tell Herb, who, while denying the possibility of the side effect, was his usual indifferent self. Take it, don't take it. He didn't really care one way or the other. So I just quit, went cold turkey, and after a few days, I felt as if I had been cured of whatever I had. The medicine was making me far, far sicker than the illness, and I dreaded that this was a preview of the chemotherapy that was about to begin.

Before I went for the port installation (it sounded like something at the Naval Academy), I decided I had to break my news to Dexter Farnham, the one non-family member I had to let in on my secret. Even though he had been a total mensch and stand-up friend about letting me continue my surgery with him when he found out I had NHL, I did worry how he would feel now that my lymphoma had gone aggressive. I wouldn't have blamed him for cutting me loose; after all, I could be bad for business, a medical Typhoid Mary. He had given me two great years, gotten me invited to speak at medical conferences around the world, validated me with his "By Appointment to His Majesty, Dexter Farnham" seal of approval, and, above all, helped me continue doing what I adored most, my surgery. I had to be grateful for what I had accomplished.

But Dexter was as elegantly noble and supportive as he had been before. He insisted on examining me, palpating my nodes, exploring my neck, holding my florid head in those amazing hands of his. What a grip, what a touch. Dexter was said to have the best hands in plastic surgery, and now I knew what his colleagues meant. If I could have been healed, revival-meeting style, by the laying on of hands, Dexter was the man to do it. He was born again, and his very touch almost made this eternal skeptic a true believer. "You'll be all right," he said with the greatest authority. He knew Herb and assured me he was one of the deans of the field. He offered the backup of other world-class oncologists should I need it, but he dismissed the possibility.

Dexter insisted that I keep working. He went through a long list of prominent doctors he knew who had cancer and were still practicing full time. I was shocked at the names, shocked they shared my secret, but proud that I was now a member of this elite, though unmentionable, society. "You'll get the chemo, be back in the office the same day. It's no big deal," Dexter insisted, in his laconic, cut-to-the-chase way. Maybe not for him, I thought, a powerful guy who could have been an action movie star in a different life. But I didn't want to display my Bronx self-doubts. I wanted to be Big Sky, Marlboro Country (minus the cigarettes) just like Dexter. So I took a deep breath and summoned up my strength to go into the chemo battle. I have to admit that Dexter's unwavering support and confidence gave me more courage than any texts I read, and certainly far more than any of the doctors who would be treating me.

The port surgery went fine, except it was weird having this tube under my collar. It made me feel fragile. I was glad I was in LA, with all its elbow room, and not in New York, where a close encounter on the subway or in Times Square could have ripped the tube out of my chest, or caused serious damage. Nor was the chemo as toxic as I had thought. Emboldened by Dexter's exhortations, and wanting to get back to the office right away, I decided to forego the anti-nausea medicine, Zofran, that always preceded a chemo session and required an hour and a half drip before the chemo could even be started. So I played tough guy, said, "Nausea is for sissies," and somehow never got nauseated. I took my first week of chemo off from the office, imagining I'd be too wiped out to do anything but curl up in a ball and be ill. But Dexter was right. I was up and rarin' to go back to my patients.

My chemo would start each morning at nine and last two hours. The "chemo lounge" at Cedars had twenty large reclining chairs where my fellow cancer fighters would be getting their drips, many into ports like mine. I never saw anyone I knew, thank goodness, and I never made any new friends in the lounge. It wasn't a bonhomie, or even bonding, sort of place. Some people were old, some very young, some dismally frail, some as healthy looking as horses. Everyone kept to himself, reading magazines, or just looking out into space. Some people brought cookies, or sometimes awful-smelling snacks—burritos, pastrami sandwiches, fried noodles, hardly breakfast fare—that seemed as if it would cause more distress than the chemo. I would think to myself, you can get through this. So I just lay back in my easy chair and let the poison drip slowly into my veins. And then I left and went back to work, just as in the good old days BC, Before Cancer. My only concession to my illness was not to do surgery on chemo days. Otherwise, I just led my life.

It was amazing to me that it was so uneventful. If I weren't getting violently sick, I worried, maybe the chemo wasn't working. Then, almost as if the god, or devil, as it were, of medicine was responding to me, I developed a strange side effect, that of extreme agitation and nervousness. I called Herb, who wrote it off as chemo beginner's jitters. So then I looked up Fludarabine in my *Physicians' Desk Reference*, and there it was as a common side effect: agitation and nervousness. I hadn't noticed it the first time because I was looking for the big stuff, aplastic anemia, cardiomyopathy, the things that kill you. Why Herb thought I wouldn't look it up was beyond me; why he didn't acknowledge the symptom was beyond the beyond. It shook my confidence in him, but I wrote it off to de minimis, little things. I didn't confront Herb, but rather gritted my teeth, thanked God that this was the only side effect, and stayed the course.

I became something of a chemo addict. One aspect of the treatment was that the Fludarabine caused a drop in all my white blood cells, not just the lymphocytes that were causing the disease. The body needs white blood cells to fight infection, and if the WBC count gets too low, the chemo must be stopped until the count comes up again. Raising the count is a medical miracle accomplished by a drug called Neupogen, which stimulates the bone marrow to produce more cells. The first time this happened, and one of my endless blood tests showed a WBC deficiency and my chemo was cut off, I felt like a junkie in need of a fix.

I got my first shot of Neupogen and came back the next day to continue the chemo, but the nurses said no. My WBC remained too low. I freaked out. I called Herb and basically begged him for the Fludarabine, my precious elixir of life. Herb drew a hard line. He said I was at risk for a life-threatening infection. I needed more WBCs. I hated Herb worse than prisoners hate their evil guards. I felt he was torturing me, not keeping me alive. I was being totally irrational, of course, but cancer isn't necessarily the stuff of reason. Fortunately, after my next Neupogen shot, my WBC went up and I was able to get my Fludarabine "fix." Luckily my blood count didn't drop below the acceptable level again. But my anxiety at getting my daily WBC test results was greater than waiting for my SAT scores at Bronx Science.

Eventually the damn treatment began to work. The rash over my face and chest began to subside. My scalp ceased aching, and my hair actually stopped falling out. Best of all, the lumps in my groin were disappearing. I was a walking miracle of science. I thus approached my work not as a form of denial and avoidance, but as a gift of life. I couldn't have been more excited to drive to East Los Angeles and help all these new immigrants realize their health and their dreams. I loved doing my surgeries. I loved working with Dexter and being at the forefront of my field. I loved being alive. And then the FBI showed up.

It was now July 1997. I had begun the chemo six months before. I was feeling lucky for the first time in my life. Karen and I had just gotten back from a wonderful trip to a facial plastic surgery meeting at the Waldorf Astoria in New York, where I was one of the stars at the gathering, aided in no small part by being Dexter Farnham's emissary. Then Karen and I went on a wonderful history, garden, and antiquing excursion to Charleston, South Carolina, and Savannah, Georgia, where I easily imagined Karen in a hoopskirt and crinolines, pouring mint juleps on the verandah of the plantation. She had just finished reading John Berendt's *Midnight in the Garden of Good and Evil* and was fascinated by the Southern eccentricities he described lurking beneath the charm and gentility. All we got was the charm. And then the FBI showed up soon after we returned. Because I first discovered that my NHL had gone aggressive on the trip to Virginia, and the lawmen descended after our trip to the Carolina Low Country, I began getting superstitious about crossing the Mason-Dixon Line. I haven't been back to the South since, much as I loved it.

It was a good thing I had a lawyer in the family, in the person of Gail's husband. Even though his specialty was corporate law, he was connected to all the captains of the local bar. Over one of Mimi's solidarity dinners, Lee had only two words for me: Larry Carmen. Larry Carmen. I'll never forget that name, as if it were a mantra. Larry

Carmen. If Melvin Belli in San Francisco was the "king of torts," Larry Carmen in Beverly Hills was the "emperor of crime," Lee rhapsodized. Did I really need an emperor of crime to handle what seemed to be a minor administrative matter about billing? Wasn't that overkill?

"It's the goddamned FBI, Alvin," Lee scolded me. "How minor can it be? Overkill? Better you kill them than they kill you."

Even though I was a frequent expert witness for lawyers and insurance companies in personal injury and workers compensation cases, I didn't have a lawyer of my own, and had never really thought about getting one. The lawyers I had dealt with liked me a lot. I was considered to be a true expert backed not only by knowledge and training but also by an active practice. I was considered to be totally objective and was hired by plaintiffs and defendants in equal measure. One of the most memorable medical legal cases I encountered involved the renowned case of Rodney King, the African American man who was stopped by the police after leading them on a long chase, and whose name has become nearly synonymous with police brutality and the LA riots of 1992. Rodney was 6'4" and very muscular. He was also very drunk. When the police told him to put his hands up, he started laughing and making jokes and waving to the helicopters that were flying overhead. This infuriated the police. Saying they felt frightened by King, they beat him up in full force.

That night was to change many people's lives in Los Angeles, lamentably for the worse. King had sustained multiple facial injuries, including a significantly displaced cheekbone and eye orbit. The entire beating was videotaped by an onlooker, whose footage was soon broadcast around the nation and world, making this a very high profile case. The case was sent to me. I assembled a team of four surgeons, including myself. We performed a six hour operation on King to reconstruct his shattered face. The surgery was successful and I had my Andy Warhol fifteen minutes of fame, as I suddenly was in demand and appeared on every major and local TV station, radio station and newspaper. I was Dr. Alvin Reiter, Rodney King's plastic surgeon. I was also asked to be the regular broadcast doctor for a local Los Angeles TV station. I declined this continuing spotlight, much to Karen's dismay; she was so proud of her husband, "doctor to kings."

Yes, the lawyers did like me, but I had had no use for them in my private life. For my house purchase I had let my broker handle everything. I didn't even have a will, which may have been a matter of denial given my illness, but it also reflected my negative feelings about the legal profession, which I saw as extremely avaricious and about as un-humanitarian as could be. Law, at least Beverly Hills law, was all about money, getting money from the studios, getting money from rich spouses, getting money from once beloved and now despised business partners. The idea of criminal law had never even crossed my mind. Wasn't that the province of drug dealers and insider traders?

"They love white-collar crime," Lee went on, doing his best to scare me into seeing Larry Carmen, for whom Lee had once worked as a summer law clerk while he was at UCLA. "Gives them class, those G-men. One Roxbury Drive doctor's worth fifty Colombian cocaine runners. Think of the publicity."

And I did. Just what I needed. Cancer-afflicted Beverly Hills Plastic Surgeon Implicated in Billing Fraud Scandal. I was glad my discussion with Lee took place out of earshot of Karen, outside under a jacaranda tree.

"Just go see Larry," Lee said. "He'll blow them right out, scare them to death. When they see who's repping you, they'll run for the hills."

149

"But he'll charge a fortune," I protested. "Medellin cartel prices."

"You get what you pay for. Don't be pennywise and pound foolish, Alvin," Lee chided me. "All you've got is your reputation. You've got to be above reproach. You're in the FBI loop. Sure, it's unfair. Sure, you did nothing. But you're in the system somehow, and you've got to get out. You have to fight fire with an extinguisher!"

So I set up a date to meet Larry Carmen. Karen pushed me to do it as well. She totally respected her brother-in-law and his legal acumen, which had made him a rich and successful man. "If Lee says go, go." So I went.

The court of the emperor was on Wilshire near Doheny in a building that indeed looked like a turreted gray castle; it lacked only a moat and a drawbridge. The office was as impenetrable as a fortress. The doors were made of steel and were tightly locked, and security cameras ringed the premises. I noticed bars on all the windows, both on the first and second floors. I waited for nearly five minutes pressing a buzzer outside before I was asked to identify myself. Finally, I was buzzed in.

Larry Carmen's wife had a local catering company, legendary for its theme parties, and her influence was apparent. Here the theme was pre-Revolutionary France, Louis XV in his après moi le deluge wretched excess. I had never seen so many antiques, statues, gilded mirrors, and other expensive bric-a-brac, and fake Titians and Rembrandts. I thought most of it was in terrible taste. But I was here for law, not aesthetics, though I thought it odd that the reading matter in the waiting room was *Art and Antiques* and *Country Life*, not the *Harvard Law Review* or even *Crime and Punishment*. I wondered how the drug dealers felt when they came in here.

I was even more taken aback by Larry Carmen. The emperor was Napoleonic in size, a tiny, dark, glowering bald man in his late fifties.

The antique desk he presided from was placed on a raised platform in the center of the room. I sat in a leather chair nearly a foot below him. Walls of law books surrounded us, and there were gold-embossed editions of those Larry Carmen had authored. There was no doubt that I was in the presence of a great authority. For such a little powerhouse, I was surprised at how weak and fishy Larry Carmen's handshake was. Maybe he didn't want to get too close to the miscreants he represented. I had thought being Lee's family I would get a warm welcome. But there was no small talk, no feeling each other out for mutual acquaintances or interests. He made me feel like a common criminal.

"There's a big campaign against insurance fraud in plastic surgery in Southern California," Carmen said, with a trace of what sounded like a New York borough accent, though I didn't dare venture out loud that perhaps we were both home boys from the Bronx. He had gleaned his information from his contacts in the U.S. Attorney's Office. I had been caught up in the net. Dexter Farnham was the big fish they were after, Larry told me, but they would take as many minnows as they could find.

"But I didn't do anything," I insisted.

Carmen just gave me a that's-what-they-all-say look. To him, I was guilty until proven innocent. He asked me a battery of questions, mostly about how much money I made. He couldn't believe that I let Dexter do the billing for the surgeries I did for him, nor that I trusted Dexter's accounting.

"Do you realize how much money you could be losing?" Carmen asked, bearing down on me incredulously. Not only had I placed myself in legal jeopardy by wearing blinders in the matter of accounting, but, worse in Carmen's mind, I wasn't making all I could.

"I have lymphoma!" I declared. "The money doesn't matter to me. All I care about is the work."

Carmen just stared at me with a cocked eyebrow. "You're a Beverly Hills plastic surgeon, Dr. Reiter. Please."

"Mr. Carmen," I said. I didn't feel comfortable calling him Larry, nor did he suggest it. "Having cancer really makes you reevaluate your priorities. I love surgery. I hate bookkeeping. Life's too short, and mine's a lot shorter."

"Cancer is no excuse," he responded. "Not for participating in a fraud."

"I didn't participate," I insisted. I wanted to walk out, but I was too dumbfounded by his icy hostility. I was riveted to my low chair.

"You did surgery on those Mexicans. You got paid. That's participation. Ignorance of the center's billing practices is no excuse. I don't care if you have a terminal brain tumor."

"How do we even know Dexter did anything wrong?" I asked him. Dexter Farnham, I wanted to say, was the Larry Carmen of plastic surgery. " He doesn't need the money…"

"Don't be naïve, Dr. Reiter."

"Maybe I am, but to my knowledge, he bills like every other doctor."

"A lot of doctors may be going down," Carmen said ominously. "The government likes this case a lot, from what I hear." He brought up the HIPPA law (Health Insurance Portability and Accountability Act) that had just been enacted, resulting from the Kennedy-Kassebaum legislation. The fraud provisions of the act, which were only a few paragraphs out of hundreds of pages of other provisions, were what had set the FBI in action, even though that action may not have been what the law intended. The way most doctors I knew had seen it, if they noticed it at all, was that it was designed to curtail obvious large-scale Medicare and Medicaid abuses, amounting to billions of dollars, not to challenge widespread mainstream billing procedures. Larry Carmen didn't care that the lawmen might be running amok. Amok was what he lived for. "They've got a new law, they need cases," he said, nearly licking his chops at the prospect of battle. "The government's hungry. Hungry for blood."

"The government loses, too, Mr. Carmen, thanks to you."

It was the only time in our meeting that the flicker of a smile illuminated his saturnine countenance. "This will take a lot of investigation. A lot, a lot..." He let the notion hang in the air. "I'll have to put some of my top people on it. We can start with a retainer of fifty thousand, against hourly billing. Of course if we go to trial it will be on a different—"

"Trial?" I interjected. "I thought this was just a subpoena to appear before a grand jury. I thought they were after Dexter Farnham. He's my friend. I wanted to help..."

"Help yourself, Dr. Reiter," the emperor decreed, cocking his eyebrow again. The notion of friendship seemed like an affront to the man's jaded intelligence. I didn't question the retainer, or try to bargain. How do you bargain with legal royalty? I thought Herb, like most oncologists, in fact, was bad in not giving me any hope or encouragement. Herb had the warmth and love of Jesus Christ Himself compared to Larry Carmen.

"What the hell did you expect, a faith healer?" Lee attacked me when I asked him to find me another lawyer. "Larry's like Metternich," Lee said, showing off his historical allusions. "He's all about realpoliitik, not making you feel good. Wanna feel good? Go to AA. Wanna stay out of jail? Stick with Larry."

First trial, now jail. The stakes got higher with every conversation. All I wanted to do was get my chemotherapy and do my surgery. I didn't want trials and jails and the FBI. I was a doctor, not a felon, but these lawyers were making me feel like a fugitive. I knew now why I avoided having a lawyer. I wished to heaven I could avoid it now. But Lee scared me, and Lee scared Karen, and Karen, who was a big believer in top credentials and always getting the best, whether doctors, lawyers, or antique dealers, insisted that I write out the fifty thousand dollar check and pay our way out of this new nightmare. And I did.

When I told Dexter I had retained Larry Carmen, he put his powerful arm around my shoulder to congratulate me. "Damn. I should have thought of him. He's the top. Watch those Feds scatter now," he assured me, and it felt good. Dexter told me that his lawyer, Roland Greene, was a close friend of Larry Carmen, and that they would make a formidable team. Greene was known for getting rich Beverly Hills murderers off the hook, men who strangled their wives, women who poisoned their husbands, kids who slaughtered their parents when they drew the line at a BMW and not a Ferrari. At least I could take comfort in the fact that I was in good, if not kind, legal hands.

Lee assured me that not only would Carmen take care of things, but that the wheels of justice turned so slowly that it would be months, if not years, before I would ever have to face the grand jury, if ever at all. I therefore would not wait for the law, which was like waiting for Godot. I would go back to my old life, which was a new life, but better than a life on trial.

Meanwhile, however, I had a new medical problem to deal with, a second cancer. A few months before, I had noticed a small bump on the tip of my nose. I assumed it was part of the lymphoma rash, but now that my face was returning to normal, the nodule on my nose remained red and began to bleed whenever I touched it. I self-diagnosed it as a basal cell carcinoma, which was the mildest form of skin cancer, slow to grow yet still capable of great disfigurement, especially on the face. One of the side effects of chemo lowers your immune system, and you are consequently more susceptible to all diseases, including skin cancer. I was glad it wasn't a squamous cell carcinoma, or a malignant melanoma, which are far more rapidly invasive, and potentially lethal. I had enough lethal for right now.

Because it was literally as plain as the nose on my face, I wanted to get the best skin cancer specialist who would do the least damage to my appearance, which in the case of a facial plastic surgeon is a very important consideration. The name that came up most frequently was Ted Kram, a professor at UCLA who specialized in a technique called Mohs microsurgery, a process in which the doctor does as little damage to the patient's skin as possible by taking off small increments of tissue over several hours, then testing the margins of the skin to make sure all the cancer has been removed. I had been trained in Mohs and had done it many times, but naturally I couldn't operate on myself. I wanted the best alter ego, and Ted Kram seemed to be the man.

Arriving for my appointment, I thought I had accidentally wandered into a bus terminal. I had never seen so many patients jammed into an office. Some were sitting on tables, others sprawled on the floor. Somehow, however, the line moved quickly, and I was in to see the doctor in less than an hour, far less time than I had anticipated. Ted was a tall, wiry character who spoke like lightning. No wonder the patients moved so quickly. With a clogged waiting room like his, I didn't expect a personal touch, and I didn't get it. He took a quick look at my nose, confirmed my diagnosis as a basal cell, but took a tiny sample for a pro forma biopsy and scheduled surgery in several weeks.

I had noted that Ted was a dermatologist, but not a plastic surgeon. Whenever I had done Mohs on a sensitive feature of my patients' faces, I would immediately follow the cancer excision with plastic surgery so as not to leave a crater or a major scar. I asked Ted if we should get a plastic surgeon in with him to patch up my nose. He looked at me as if I wanted to get Michael Jordan to help me with my backyard basketball game. Talk about overkill, he said, ridiculing my suggestion. "It's nothing. Tiny. Miniscule. I'll take care of it." He machine gunned the words, making a knitting needle motion with his miniscule hands, which, I noticed, were beautifully manicured. His total self-confidence had convinced me enough to go against my own practice of getting plastic surgery on the cancer site. I had enough problems in my life at this point. I guess I just hoped that these elegant hands would work the magic everyone said they did. Who was I to argue with the reputation of this Beverly Hills doctor, not to mention a standing-room only waiting room? All the shocks to my system had made me overly sensitive, and I reassured myself that I was just being paranoid.

I didn't question my decision until one night at a mahjong game Karen hosted in our "Chinese" room (the room was appointed with Oriental rugs, cherrywood furniture, exquisite silks, an ancestors' shrine, and an elaborate seventeenth-century marquetry veneered commode. Karen would serve jasmine tea and let the sounds of Chinese opera fill the air). One guest, Sarah, the wife of a distinguished ocular surgeon, somehow noticed the lump on my nose, and didn't mince words in telling me to take care of it. She was outspoken, but she always meant well, so I didn't hold her abrasive style against her. However, when I mentioned that Ted Kram was going to remove the nodule, Sarah went way beyond abrasive. "That butcher!" she shrieked. "You cannot go to him. He'll destroy your face. Cancel first thing tomorrow."

Karen's mahjong party didn't seem the right place to debate the skills of Ted Kram, but Sarah wouldn't let it go and basically ruined an enchanted evening. Karen had heard of Ted, nothing bad, but she trusted my judgment, and my judgment was that Ted was a super-skilled professional. So we ignored Sarah's alarming attack, writing it off to perhaps something personal between Sarah's husband and Ted. We didn't look further. We had enough to worry about beside the tip of my nose. Besides, I had lymphoma, Stage IV, end of line. Wasn't it a little vain, or hubristic, to split hairs over my nose when my body was hanging by a thread? I wasn't exactly superstitious, but I was reluctant to push my luck by making a big fuss over my nose.

I went for the surgery by myself. It seemed minor, and I wanted to spare Karen the mob in the waiting room, and the wait itself, which could be quite long with Mohs. As it turned out, the surgery was like the lightning round on *Wheel of Fortune*. I wasn't even given a gown. Ted came into the small operating room followed by about ten students, who made the surgery seem like the fifties prank where kids would see how many people they could jam into a phone booth. Ted was rushed and distracted. He sent me out into the waiting room until the next round of excision without even putting a dressing on the wound, only a little Band-Aid. Blood began dripping all over my shirt and jacket, and a nurse slapped another Band-Aid on.

There were three more rounds, until Ted announced he had it all. There was a huge hole, but before I could question it, he rapidly began sewing it up. During this reconstructive phase, Ted didn't even give me any sedation, as I did my patients. He just injected some topical anesthetic, which didn't stop the pain of his procedure. Only after my anguished protests did he inject some more. And then some more. Finally, he completed his stitching and stuck a thick dressing over it. He had spent no more than a total of a half hour with me, if that. "Piece of cake," he declared, and sent me home.

I looked like Jack Nicholson after Roman Polanski had tried to slice off his nose for being nosy in *Chinatown*. Karen thought I looked cute. She assured me the great Ted Kram had to know what he was doing, and that I should stop worrying. But a few days afterward I noticed through the loosening bandages that the skin was black and necrotic, or dead, and the wound was infected. It wasn't just dried blood. I was shocked and insisted on going back to Ted on an emergency basis, which put me ahead of the long queue at his bakery of skin. Ted took a look and said to come back in three months.

I ended up having to clean and treat my own wound infection. It took many months to heal, and I was left with an unsightly scar on my nose. I told my patients I had a basal cell. I had no choice; it was right there. Too much tennis, I quipped. They must have thought I was the most country club doctor in Beverly Hills. First the red face, which I wrote off to sunburn, now my tennis-obsessed nose. You could fess up to skin cancer, but not lymphoma. Still, I felt embarrassed and unsightly. Lionel Barrymore, known as "The Great Profile," I could no longer be. Now it was more like Captain Hook.

I was furious at Ted Kram, and at myself for not following my better instincts to enlist a plastic surgeon. Cancer can cloud your judgment, to say the least. When I saw Ted's bill to my health insurance company, I flipped. Eight thousand dollars for a half hour? I asked to see his operative notes. What made the bill so huge was Ted's charging for a complicated muscle skin flap reconstructive procedure. The catch was that there was no muscle on the nose. He didn't do that at all. What he did do was simply pull the skin across the wound under so much pressure that the skin ripped apart, causing the necrosis and ultimate unsightliness.

Ted Kram had committed what I felt was clear medical fraud, right on me, and I didn't see the FBI going after him. But I wasn't a rat, and wasn't going to expose this so-called colleague, even though he had disfigured me and was getting rich in the process. Ted Kram was a member of one of the august bodies that oversaw all doctors in the Golden State. A few months later I happened to treat a patient whose wife had been Ted's office manager for years. When I mentioned that Ted had done, or rather butchered, my still festering nose, he chuckled about how Ted "took liberties" with his billing. The laugh was on me.

My nose may have been bad, but the rest of my body was looking better. The redness was almost gone. The lumps in my groin were imperceptible. The chemo seemed to be working. But I wouldn't know for sure until I had another CAT scan, as well as a PET scan, in which radioactive glucose would be injected into my veins to locate areas of high metabolism, and hence more rapidly dividing, i.e., cancerous, cells. Looks were always potentially deceiving. Besides, with the FBI and Ted Kram's hatchet job, I certainly wasn't feeling lucky. This time I went for my scans at night. The bowels of Cedars-Sinai after-hours is a spooky place indeed. It feels like a morgue. And the PET scan machine is the closest thing to a waking coffin in modern medicine.

During the light of a busy day, you have enough distractions to keep your mind off mortality, but in the dead of night, inside this high-tech coffin, that's all you can think about. The lugubrious atmosphere wasn't aided by the lab tech, who didn't utter a word throughout the seemingly endless hour or so the scan lasted. At the end, I threw all caution to the wind and asked him how it looked, knowing full well there wasn't a chance in hell of his telling me. I was resigned to wait the agonizing day, or two, or maybe three, to get the news from Herb.

After a long silence, the tech shocked me totally by uttering the nicest phrase I ever heard, "It looks good to me." I didn't press him on it, but I did give him a big hug. I'm not sure what he thought about this public display of affection, but, well, who was there to see it? Besides, I couldn't control myself. The joy was that powerful. Then the tech, stunned by my happiness, breached all protocol by letting me see the X-ray pictures. He pointed out how there was no cancer. I remember on my first scan how bleak my cancer-ridden insides looked in black and white. Now that same black and white looked like glorious Technicolor to me, with Cinemascope and Stereophonic Sound thrown in. What a magic sense of relief! It was as if the tech and I were the only people on earth, there in that creepy Cedars basement. Actually there were three of us: me, the tech, and those sheets of plastic without a trace of cancer.

I went home to a late-night celebration with Karen. "I guess I'll have to put up with you for a little longer," she said, before giving me a big kiss. She gathered our cats around us. "I don't really care that much," she joked, "but Doodle and Wojge and Tinker and Dexter, you guys are overjoyed, aren't you? Let's celebrate with some catnip, while

160

you tell us about your CAT scan. Here's to your good health, Daddy. Meow!" Karen and I had never been closer. We made the tenderest love that night, a victory celebration of my battle with cancer.

When I finally met with Herb, he confirmed all the good news. The chemo was over. I was in remission. Of course, party pooper that he was, Herb had to warn me that it could come roaring back at any time, and that I would have to come back for scans every year.

Happiness wasn't in Herb's lexicon, so I didn't want to seem too happy and bring sunshine to his always rained-out parade. But I left his office with a big smile, ready to take the world on with all the vigor of a young vital surgeon, a healer who had been healed. I had completely forgotten about the FBI. No news had been good news. I suppose in the back of my mind I assumed that by giving that blood money to the vampire Larry Carmen I had bought my way out of an unpleasant spot, just as I might buy my way out of coach and into business class. Oh well, that was only money, and I was glad I had enough not to care. Besides it was a small price for peace of mind. I had to get back to my life, my wonderful life. I had saved my own life, and now I had others to help. Little did I know at that blissful moment who that most significant other was going to be.

Chapter Seven

LA LAW

Even though my being in remission had given me a new lease on life, I didn't have a great deal of confidence that the lease would be that long. Accordingly, when my landlord on Roxbury Drive demanded that I sign a new ten-year lease on my office, at an extortionately increased Beverly Hills rent, I had to refuse. I was cautious about being too cocky, and ten years would have been cocky indeed. However, I hated to give up my prime location, so I downsized into the only space available in the building, a windowless closet of an office that was nearly as claustrophobic as the PET scan that had set me free. Going from 2,000 square feet to 600 required me to give up most of the amenities of my old space: the plants, the fish tank, the extra examining suites. It wasn't my choice; I had to be practical.

Not that my practice was booming. During my chemotherapy, I had stopped doing any surgery during my treatment week, and during the rest of the month I did far less than I had before I had gotten sick. Before cancer, I had been a real go-getter, a networker, meeting other doctors, doing emergency calls, working the teaching hospital circuit, all of which brought in patients. After cancer, I followed the path of least resistance and relied on Dexter to funnel me nearly all my surgery patients. I just didn't have the moxie at that point to hustle for business. Besides, it wasn't the business that thrilled me; it was the surgery. Meanwhile, my regular ENT patients kept coming in. I was glad my red face had cleared up, and even gladder when my hacked-off nose healed as well, so I didn't have anything to apologize for except my cramped new quarters. Beverly Hills doctors are expected to put on a big show, to live beyond their means, to keep up grand appearances. I was torn between that glamorous territorial imperative and the reality of living, not within my means, but within my lifetime. I told my patients the new space, or lack thereof, was temporary.

Just as I was adjusting to my new quarters, and planning to resume surgery full time, I got a call from Larry Carmen. His sepulchral voice, the voice of doom, commanded me to come to his office. It was early 1998. I hadn't heard from him for months, and I had thought he had made his calls, pulled his strings, and made a bad dream go away. But then I remembered Lee's admonition about how slowly the wheels of justice turned, and I suddenly realized that the possibility of being caught under those grinding wheels was very real, especially when the imperial rasp of Larry Carmen announced, "This is urgent."

I arrived at the castle and went through all the security checks before the multiple doors were unbarred. The first order of business from his exalted throne was to tell me that I had used up my retainer, and that he needed another $35,000. His fee was $500 an hour; the junior partner on my case, Rich Feig, whom Carmen always referred to as "my Yale man" because he had gone to Yale Law School with the Clintons, was billed out at $400. It added up quickly, with both of them sitting in. Carmen told me how many investigators he had on the case, and how much they had learned about the Beverwil Surgery Center, and, bottom line, none of it was good. In fact, it was awful. My revered Dexter Farnham, according to Larry Carmen and his team of sleuths, was running a total Ali-Baba-Den-of-Thieves operation.

Larry proudly presented me with a huge, costly pile of investigative dossiers on the center, its employees, its doctors, its patients. He threw out a few tidbits. All the other surgeons who worked at the center, men I assumed were pillars of our field, had skeletons in their closets. One was a recovering cocaine addict, another an alcoholic, a third had served time for insider trading. I had cancer. Dexter had assembled a "dirty dozen" cadre of flawed physicians whose flaws would make them beholden to him. Dexter himself was richer than I had ever imagined, richer than Croesus, investment banker rich, not doctor rich. He had secret accounts Carmen's team had unearthed in Singapore, the Caymans, Anguilla, Switzerland. He had secret safes in the office, and secret bag men who came to the center late at night to take the money away, far, untraceably far, away. There were a lot of secrets.

And all this money, millions upon millions, was coming from the noses and eyelids and breasts and stomachs and thighs of Mexicans and El Salvadoreans and Vietnamese and Thais and a veritable United Nations of "new" Americans who wanted the American Dream of Beverly Hills plastic surgery. When I did the surgery on these patients, I had no idea about their financial situation or their health insurance. The East Los Angeles office manager, Ramon Cruz, who was Dexter's Latin major domo, did all the translations, all the payments, all the forms. I was at a distinct disadvantage not speaking the language. I just did the work. It wasn't a classic doctor-patient relationship. But those relationships were a thing of a honeyed past, of Currier and Ives prints, of house calls, of Norman Rockwell portraits depicting avuncular family doctors examining angelic little children. Today was the day of the HMO, of anonymity. There was no interchange to be had, just work to do, which I gratefully did. It worked fine for a doctor with cancer.

But now, according to Carmen, Ramon had disappeared, as had many key records of the center. I didn't know about the records, but I had been told Ramon had gone home to Costa Rica to aid his ailing mother. Carmen sneered. "Ailing mother! You really believe that?"

"I don't see why not."

"Can't you see what's going on there?" he asked, clearly annoyed.

"I'm a doctor, not Sherlock Holmes. Not Liz Smith. I'm not interested in gossip," I replied, attempting to defend myself. "Why should I assume the worst?"

"Because the worst is about to happen to you, doctor." Larry Carmen told me how he had been successful in postponing my grand jury summons, but that, in the process, the government had learned more and more, and worse and worse about the center, and the scope of its case had expanded. "You're not a witness, doctor," Larry boomed at me. "You're a target." As were all Dexter Farnham's crack team of Beverly Hills surgeons, breast men and face men and nose men and eye men, super-successful men with flaws and pasts I had no reason to know about.

"A target? What does that mean?" I didn't like the ominous sound of the word.

"It could mean prison. Five years. Ten. The end of your good life as you know it. The U.S. Attorney really likes this case. Really likes it." The emperor smacked his lips.

"Well, how have you handled cases like this before?"

"There haven't been cases like this before," Carmen said.

Then why didn't you tell me this fifty thousand dollars ago, I thought to myself. I thought he was an expert.

"This is new ground," the Yale man chimed in, as if reading my doubts, citing the newly created HIPAA act. "We can make new law here."

At my expense, I thought but didn't say.

"Nobody's gone after high-class medical fraud before. This is untilled soil," Carmen said. I thought of Ted Kram's $8,000 half hour butchery, where a highly credentialed and certified doctor blatantly fabricated a bill for a complex procedure he never intended to do. Creative billing indeed. Apparently many doctors did the same thing, especially plastic surgeons, where the line between functional and cosmetic could be very, very thin.

The only doctor I could recall who had ever gotten into any trouble, and his trouble was with an insurance company, not the FBI, was a neighbor of mine, Ivan Barrow, an ocular plastic surgeon who lived in one of Bel Air's grandest mansions and drove a British racing green Aston Martin like the one James Bond careened about in *Goldfinger*. Barrow was an assembly line doctor on a line that moved as fast as his Aston Martin. He would do five surgeries a day; his patients all went in with some sort of visual impairment, and somehow all went out looking beautiful. And none of them ever paid a penny for it.

One day, one of the insurance companies put two and two together and went after Barrow. The company wanted to get its money back. This was elective plastic surgery, it insisted, and was not covered by them; it was not vision repair, which was. But Barrow and his team of lawyers contacted all his patients and prepped them well. When the insurance investigators contacted them, every single patient—and there were hundreds— held the line that they had problems with their eyesight, not their looks. I suppose the patients were afraid that the insurance company was going to take the money out of their pockets if they were in on the scheme. Not one patient ratted out Barrow, and the insurance company was completely stymied and went down in a rare defeat. Barrow bought a new Ferrari to celebrate his triumph.

The one ray of hope, Larry Carmen noted, was that none of the Latina and Asian patients that his investigators had contacted had shown any inclination to break ranks with Dexter's doctors. All said that they loved their surgery, that they were physically sick before and were feeling better now.

"But the FBI's just warming up," the Yale man cautioned. "They'll find some malcontents to testify."

A malcontent, I learned, was what had triggered the entire investigation. Marta, a long-term secretary in the East LA office, had been viciously teased for being fat by the recently departed Ramon. Dexter had done lipo on her several times, but afterward, she always ate the weight back on, and even Dexter, the forgiving man of Christ, mercilessly harangued her about her churro and Oreo addiction. I knew Marta, and I liked her because she was smart and efficient. Karen, who had a natural empathy for anyone with a weight problem, introduced Marta to Weight Watchers and took her to months of meetings.

But nothing worked. Marta simply couldn't stop eating junk, and Dexter (and his lieutenant Ramon) couldn't stand having someone up front who was such a terrible advertisement. The master of beauty was appalled that this woman could not master her appetites, and he constantly let her have it. Not only were Marta's feelings battered. She was a jealous type to begin with, with Beverly Hills aspirations and consumption patterns, loving to shop at the sales at Saks and Neiman Marcus, always buying sizes she could never fit into. She hated seeing all the newly skinny patients, especially because, unlike herself, they stayed skinny. Eventually, her bitter attitude got her fired, and apparently hell had no fury like a fat employee scorned by a plastic surgeon.

Ironically, Ramon was one of the most unattractive men I had ever seen: sloppy, obese, with a deeply recessive chin. I was surprised that Dexter tolerated such lack of discipline, and that Dexter hadn't operated on Ramon himself. But Ramon seemed exempt from Dexter's impossible standards. I assumed it was because Ramon had single-handedly recruited and managed all the immigrant business. But according to Larry Carmen, Dexter was bound to Ramon because Ramon had too much on him. He knew where all Dexter's figurative bodies were buried; he had buried them himself. And now he was a fugitive from justice.

I still didn't buy any of it. Dexter was still a giant, a god, and, most of all, a friend to me. Marta had an axe to grind, and the government had cases to make, so why not try to bring down a god? But I'd still bet on the god. I hated bureaucrats, I hated red tape, I hated busybodies and snoops and rats. It all smacked to me of Nazi Germany or Stalinist Russia, Big Brother watching you. Dexter, and I, and all the doctors at Beverwil, were simply practicing our duties as doctors. Let the FBI go after the real criminals, the destroyers and stealers, not the healers. I thus paid Larry Carmen $35,000 more in blood money, just to make the hassles go away so I could concentrate on the things that mattered.

I did, however, begin to look more closely at the center as I worked there. How could I not? My curiosity had been piqued by the horrific allegations. I didn't see much. Everyone was on good behavior. The investigation was never, ever mentioned by anyone in Dexter's orbit, doctors or staff. There was a total blackout on gossip. I was never much on office intrigues to begin with, and even less so after cancer.

Strangely enough, now that I was in remission and had the strength and the will to work, less and less business was coming my way. At one point I was only doing a handful of surgeries a week. I complained to Dexter, who insisted we drive out to his main office in suburban Monterey Park to get to the bottom of things.

We met with the new office manager, Octavio, who had replaced Ramon, during what I was still led to believe was Ramon's leave of absence. Octavio also owned a salsa club in East LA that Karen had once dragged me to both in the interest of office goodwill and because of her love of Latin culture. He was, unlike Ramon, a natty dresser and had a ready smile. Dexter spoke to Octavio in fluent Spanish, then said, insistently, "Tell him in English. Go ahead. He needs to hear it." Octavio shuffled and mumbled and looked downward before he could speak. His secretary, Luisa, sat by with a pained expression.

"Say it, Octavio," Dexter ordered him.

"Dr. Reiter…he's not the same. I'm not sure if it's his cancer, or something else, but patients…patients…"

"What patients, Octavio," Dexter prodded him impatiently.

"The patients. They just don't want to see him anymore."

I was dumbstruck, both by the comment that patients were shunning me, as well as by the fact Octavio knew my secret.

"Is that true, Luisa?" Dexter asked the secretary.

Luisa, too, didn't want to talk, nor could she address me directly. "No, sir. The patients don't feel comfortable with him. They don't like him. They don't trust him to do surgery on them."

"Why not, Luisa?" Dexter pressed her. I was "him," not "me." I was disconnected from my own life. It felt horrible.

"Maybe because he is sick."

"I'm not sick!" I insisted, raising my voice.

Dexter gave me a scornful look. "Alvin, keep your cork on," he said.

"People don't want him to operate on them. They say no. They go somewhere else," Luisa said sadly, unable to look at me.

It was a relatively silent ride back to Beverly Hills. "Well, Alvin what can I do? The customer is always right."

"But I'm the same."

"No man with cancer is ever the same. Don't delude yourself," Dexter said sharply.

"Why did you tell them?" I asked. My sense of betrayal had to be obvious to him.

"There's no secret in our office. They work for you, for me. They need to know, and they know. Listen, I can see it myself. You're too nervous. Sure, you've been through a lot. It's understandable. But you can't see yourself as others see you, and they see a doctor who doesn't give them confidence. You must go to work on getting a cooler head, Alvin. Maybe go to a workshop," Dexter suggested.

Nothing could have infuriated me more. I wasn't an addict. I didn't need twelve steps. I just wanted to work, and now I couldn't. I felt desperate, the way I did when Herb withheld my Fludarabine. Well, maybe I was an addict. I was addicted to my profession, to surgery, to life. I may have been in remission, but on that endless westbound ride back home on the Santa Monica Freeway, with Bentleys beside pickup trucks, the great LA melting pot, I felt like death warmed over. There is nothing worse for a surgeon than doubting himself, and this day had shaken my confidence like no other.

It wasn't as if the patients dried up completely, but there were fewer of them. I was deeply insulted that the patients who were rejecting me

171

were judging a book by its cover. It didn't help that I didn't speak to them in their own language. Ramon had translated for them when he had brought them in for exams. Now Octavio did it. It was surreal, the endless translations. Octavio would announce their symptoms, I'd examine them, ask questions, which Octavio would translate, and, then translate their answers back to me.

If I had been the patient I wouldn't have felt comfortable, either, but that was the price of getting a Beverly Hills doctor, and one without a price tag. This is what was driving the FBI crazy: that these people weren't being operated on in Tijuana, where the FBI probably thought they belonged, but in Beverly Hills. They were getting something for nothing, a very big something, and that was un-American in a land where you were supposed to get what you paid for. With an emphasis on pay. But that was Big Medicine today, that was the way of health insurance. If you could get a great doctor, why not. The problem for me was that I was that great doctor, and these people still didn't want me.

Another bizarre problem arose when I began receiving insurance checks, large checks in the thousands, for surgeries I had not done on patients I had never heard of. Everyone likes pennies from heaven, but I preferred to do the work. Upon further investigation, I discovered the checks were for anesthesia, not surgery. Obviously there had to be a big mistake. There was. I found out that the anesthesiologist, Jeff Cooley, had been suspended as a Blue Shield provider because he had been caught giving IV Demerol to himself while doing anesthesiology at various Los Angeles hospital operating rooms. The California Medical Board had given him a slap on the wrist and briefly suspended his license. Blue Shield was harsher than the med board; they had dropped him completely as a provider. Jeff, however, didn't want to stop working, so he put down my name as the anesthesiologist and expected me to sign these big checks over to him. As for the checks, they were two and three times the normal rate for the procedures in question, but just as Ted Kram had done with me, Jeff had trumped up the hours and the complexity so he could have windfall profits.

I immediately set up a meeting with Jeff and Dexter, which was a huge mistake. Dexter adored Jeff Cooley, who was big and rawboned and Kansan and brilliant, a man in Dexter's image. He was also a recovering drug addict like Dexter—they went to NA meetings together. That was a tie that could not be cut asunder. Also like Dexter, Jeff loved money. At Harvard, where he had played basketball, Jeff was a hippie druggie, the stoned sports star he could have never been at straight-laced Kansas State. Now the only remnant of Jeff's psychedelic past was his complete collection of Grateful Dead CDs. Jeff insisted on piping CNBC into our OR so he could hear the stock market quotes during surgery. These were the NASDAQ years of irrational exuberance, and Jeff would often duck out to call his broker. Jeff lived in a Malibu dream house, and had a collection of '60s muscle cars: GTOs, 442s, souped-up Corvairs, Shelby Cobras. He dated lots of gorgeous rock band backup singers. He was a player as well as a brilliant anesthesiologist. But I didn't want him playing with my career.

"Where's the damage?" Dexter, said, turning on me as if I had accused Jeff of child molestation.

"I'm not an anesthesiologist, and I have never given anesthesia," I protested.

"Neither am I, Alvin," Dexter said impatiently, tossing down a sheath of Blue Shield Explanation of Benefits reports. "Read them."

I did. On each of them Dexter was named as the anesthesiologist.

"Just give Jeff his checks," Dexter said, peremptorily.

"Hey, man, don't be so uptight," Jeff taunted me. "I'd do the same for you."

"I wouldn't ask," I said. "And neither did you, Jeff."

"Alvin has obviously never played on a team," Dexter said snidely.

"This is so bogus," I said. "We're in enough trouble here—"

Uh-oh! I nearly bit my tongue. I had made the forbidden comment, the ultimate faux pas. Even an oblique reference to the FBI was "negative energy," as Dexter called it. If it went unspoken, it would no longer exist, in his view.

Dexter heard it and turned beet red. He strode over to me as if he were about to slug me. Jeff stalked over as well. Each was about a foot taller than I. "There's the door, Alvin." Dexter pointed to his office door. "We're colleagues here. We're here to help each other. When you had your problems, we kept you going. Now Jeff has a problem. I know what you're thinking, Alvin, and stop being a fool. Remember. Nobody gets hurt. If you don't like it, there's the door." I had commented on several other occasions about business practices that I did not like, and in a very polite and direct way Dexter Farnham invariably told me where that door was and that there would be no hard feelings. No hard feelings? Sure. It was like bargaining with Joseph Stalin. Do or die.

Looking back, I obviously should have taken that exit strategy. But I didn't. Instead I signed over the checks to Jeff, nearly $25,000 worth. But I told them no more, exit or no exit. I never got any more. Nor did I get much more surgery. Dexter remained cordial, but my "square" response to Jeff's solution to his suspension had branded me as a spoilsport, if not a tattletale. When Karen heard the story, she told me to find somewhere else to operate. She had been off Dexter ever since she met his new wife, his fourth. Dexter had met Inga, a Barbie doll stewardess, in NA and had done every possible cosmetic procedure on her as part of his courtship. That any man could marry someone so shallow had made Karen reconsider her opinion of the great Dexter Farnham. But I couldn't hold that against him. Men were men, and flesh was weak, and plastic surgeons were often Pygmalions who couldn't stop themselves in their pursuit of beauty. No, what bothered me was not Dexter's choice of women, but the fact that Larry Carmen—and the FBI—might just have been right about him. But inertia is powerful, especially since I was still enervated by my illness. I kept hanging on, hoping the patients would be sent my way again, hoping that Dexter would remember that his mission—and his gift— was one of health and not of wealth. A few months later, I got a tearful phone call from the secretary Luisa. She had been fired, but she wasn't calling me for a reference. Instead she was calling to apologize. The story she had confirmed the day I talked to her with Dexter, that the patients had stopped wanting to see me because I was cancerous, was a fabrication. It had been made up not by Octavio, but by Dexter himself, who had written the script for Octavio and Luisa to act out. The patients still liked me, Luisa assured me. They always did. They had been asking for me, but they had been told I wasn't available. But why, I asked. Because, Luisa said, Dexter had decided I wasn't trustworthy, that I wasn't a team player.

I had no idea how manipulative Dexter could be. I had thought he was the most direct, up-front person there was. Luisa knew all the rumors about the billing fraud, though she knew no details. She did speculate that whatever was going on, if it was indeed fraudulent and

I found out, Dexter was concerned that I might blow the whistle on him. Dexter, Luisa was convinced, to my deep regret and dismay, loved money more than he loved medicine.

Further handwriting on the wall appeared with the issuance of the center's new promotional brochures. There were pictures of the state-of-the-art equipment, pictures of all the doctors next to their high-prestige bios. I appeared in the Spanish edition, but somehow was left out of the English one. It might have been an oversight, but even after I mentioned it, it was never corrected.

By fall 1998, I was getting used to the reduced scale of my practice. Still, I was grateful to be seeing patients in Beverly Hills, in my cubicle. And I continued to perform my surgical cases at the Beverwil Center. But the Monterey Park referrals basically dried up. Dexter, who was never warm in the best of times, was cordial but distant. He no longer invited me to London or Paris or New York to lecture with him. I was off the cutting edge; I would have to cut my own edge from there on. And just as I was planning to do so, Larry Carmen made another of his sepulchral calls summoning me to the castle. I assumed he wanted more retainer money, but he didn't. He and Rich Feig wanted to tell me of an offer I had to refuse. It was an offer from the U.S. Attorney's office of "transactional immunity" in an appearance before the grand jury, an appearance that Larry had postponed for over a year.

At last it was time to face the music. But now, having had my eyes opened to the realities of the center, I was far less trepidatious than I had been a year ago. I actually had something to say now. But Larry Carmen wouldn't have me say a word of it. He had already turned down the government offer, and needed my approval of his rejection as a mere formality. The year before he had turned down for me what was a quite limited grant of immunity known as "Queen for a Day." I remembered the old TV show by the same name in which a deserving woman with more than her share of misery and woe was celebrated amidst tears and cheers. For me, Queen for a Day meant that I could testify without the evidence I gave under oath being used against me. However, the government could use any other testimony by anyone else and any other evidence against me, so I was literally a protected queen only for that day. This new transactional immunity offer was the whole enchilada, from what I understood, and it was not given frequently. My ears sparked to this phrase, "transactional immunity," as it was the same deal Monica Lewinsky had just gotten to testify about her affair with President Clinton. If it was good enough for "that woman," why wasn't it good enough for me?

"Because you've got no blockbuster testimony," Carmen shouted down from his raised pedestal. "You'll only piss the government off. Then they'll come after you."

"Hey, immunity is immunity," I responded. "If I get immunity how can they come after me?"

"It's only immunity about the center," Rich Feig said.

"What else do I need immunity for? My cats?"

"It's a trick, a fishing expedition. You can only lose. If you can't hang Farnham, and you can't, they'll hang you. You have to turn it down." The emperor had issued his fiat.

"But if I turn it down..." I tried to ask.

"You will turn it down!" the emperor decreed.

"Then what next? Won't they come after me for not testifying?"

"You're calling their bluff."

Great. Just the game I wanted to play, calling the FBI's bluff. I found out that Carmen had had this offer for three weeks, and had been sitting on it without telling me. Now I had only three days left to make up my mind, but I didn't really have any choice. Carmen had made up my mind for me. He had put me in a box, a locked box. That's what emperors do to their subjects.

That day I had taken a cab to Larry Carmen's office because my car was in the shop. It was the end of the day, and Carmen made the grand gesture of offering to drive me home in his Rolls Corniche. It was an $85,000 ride home, and the most personal we had gotten in two years. When Carmen saw my house, his eyes lit up and a huge smile crossed his face. "That's a helluva house. Some house."

I didn't invite him in, but I sensed he wanted to see it all. Then he said the strangest thing. "What's more important to you, your freedom or your house?"

I didn't realize that was a choice I had to make. I never thought my freedom was in jeopardy. But before I could compose my thoughts to ask him what he meant, the emperor had laid rubber and roared away.

Karen was enormously suspicious that I wasn't taking the immunity deal. To her, immunity sounded like immunity. She didn't want me to cover for Dexter Farnham, and at this point I didn't want to either, although I really didn't know much, except I couldn't forget how shabbily he had treated me, and was angry about the team player chicanery with Jeff Cooley. It seemed like a good idea for her to call her brother-in-law for a second opinion.

Naturally, with Lee there was only one opinion: Larry Carmen was a genius. Do whatever he says. Besides, I should never be a fink and inform on my colleagues. That was the worst form a Beverly Hills doctor could display, a rat under pressure. So Karen took the law into her own hands and made an appointment to see Larry Carmen herself. It wasn't a cheap date: both Larry and Rick met with her for four hours, for a total of $900 an hour, or $3,600. Plus they charged her for three hours of "prep," another $2,700, so the consultation, or browbeating, came to $6,300—this on top of the eight hours, or $7,200, (four hours consult, four hours prep) they had billed me for our last meeting. Curiously, those $13,500 of legal fees did nothing to assuage Karen's doubts. She still thought I should take the immunity deal. But Lee did not, and in the end, I listened to what I assumed was the voice of experience, of objective in-law reason. Karen, too, didn't like going against Lee, so we continued with the Emperor of Crime.

For six months, I thought Lee had been right. I heard not a peep from the government, not a peep from Larry Carmen. I thought the FBI witch hunt was over. In late 1998 I had another PET scan that showed no evidence of active cancer. For now, I remained in complete remission. I thus remained cautiously optimistic, and worked hard at my practice, looking to replace Dexter Farnham as my source of surgery and inspiration. I rarely went to the Beverwil Center; I saw him even less. I was living fine without him, and, above all, I was living. Live and let live. For the first time in a long time, I felt slightly relaxed.

Again I remembered the Yiddish expression *kinahurra:* the idea is that you should never get too complacent, too happy, too relaxed, because the moment you do, everything will be taken away from you. I always thought of it as superstitious old-world thinking at its most primitive, yet it informed a lifetime of my behavior. Prepare for the worst, and don't exult in your successes and good fortune. Most of my Jewish friends, no matter how successful, subscribe to this grim worldview, and never stop looking over their shoulders. By now I had been in California so long that I yearned to live, metaphorically, in Pacific sunshine rather than Bronx gloom. So I began to look on the bright side. One of my New Year's resolutions of 1999 was to stop being such a pessimist and look on the bright side. Big mistake.

One evening in February, Karen and I were awakened by a blood-curdling scream. We rushed downstairs, looked around the house, and were horrified to find one of our four cats, the orange tabby Tinker, lying motionless on the floor. He was still warm, but he wasn't breathing. Karen and I rushed Tinker to the vet, who pronounced our favorite cat dead on arrival. The cause was a suspected brain aneurysm.

Tinker had been hit by a car in 1996, but I was deeply proud to have helped save his life at that point, spending hours on the phone to the veterinary department of UC Davis, to find the proper diuretic to reduce the brain swelling from the accident, something our local vet was clueless about. Tinker pulled through, but he was never again the same supercat he had been.

Named after a character on the English television series *Lovejoy*, about a charming but unscrupulous antique dealer, Tinker, before the accident, was the Arnold Schwarzenegger of cats, powerful, fearless, and very, very muscular. After the accident, Tinker became a fat cat, which upset Karen, who wanted even her pets thin. Tinker had the huge appetite Karen and I suppressed in ourselves, eating everything, and lying around like a pasha. He remained loving, and enjoyed curling up in our bed, but his old energy was spent. His head injury had led to diabetes insipidis, which caused him to drink a lot, and pee a lot. The pet shop was amazed at how much litter I would buy. Karen and I were obviously overprotective of our cats, treating them like the children we didn't have. So losing Tinker was like losing a child.

Tinker's body was kept in a refrigerator at the pet hospital until we could bring him home. We sat with him a whole day in the living room, sitting shiva. We read cat poems. And we cried. Then we bought a little casket, and put all Tinker's favorite toys in it, and buried him in our garden, our own little paradise, our own Elysian Fields. Karen's mother, Mimi, and a good friend of hers, another cat lover, came to our sad funeral. We read a particularly poignant pet poem, called "The Rainbow Bridge," which would prove to be tragically prophetic:

> There is a bridge connecting heaven and earth. It is called the Rainbow Bridge, because of its many colors. Just this side of the Rainbow Bridge is a land of meadows, hills and valleys with lush green grass. When a beloved pet dies, the pet goes to this place. There is always food and water and warm spring weather. The old and frail animals are young again. Those who are maimed are made whole again. They play all day with each other. There is only one thing missing. They are not with their special person who loved them on earth. Each day they run and play until the day comes when one suddenly stops playing and looks up. Their eyes are staring! And this one suddenly runs from the group! You have been seen, and when you and your special friend meet, you take him or her in your arms and embrace. Your face is kissed again and again, and you look once more into the eyes of your trusting pet. Then you cross the Rainbow Bridge together, never again to be separated.

When Tinker had been buried and everyone was gone, Karen got an especially glum expression on her normally glowing face. "This is a bad sign," Karen, who I used to say was part Navajo because of her uncanny ability to read the smoke signals of the future, said, "A bad sign."

I told her not to talk like that. After all, I was on a new positive kick, Mr. California, all's right with the world. It was bad enough to lose the wonderful Tinker, worse to think it meant more grim tidings.

"It's a bad sign," Karen kept saying, completely lost in her grief.

And, once again, Karen was right. Within days of Tinker's death, I got another voice-of-doom call from Larry Carmen, summoning me to the castle. He refused to tell me what he wanted. My first assumption was yet more money. This time I was wrong, dead wrong.

I brought Karen with me this time. We had paid mightily for the pleasure of Larry's company with her back in September; this time we would be there together.

Rich Feig sat by Carmen's side, saying nothing but charging a lot. The $13,500 pedestal, I thought.

"You're going to be arrested next week," Carmen intoned.

What did that mean?

"They're charging you with criminal fraud. I'm not sure how many counts, but they're charging you. I worked out a deal so they wouldn't come and get you. You go to them. You'll be released under your own recognizance pending the trial."

What about the immunity deal? I thought. What about not being charged at all, which is what that immunity deal was all about? I thought I was just a witness, a witness to Dexter's wrongdoing, to that of the other doctors at the money machine that was the Beverwil Center. I had a sense that Larry Carmen had sold me down the river, a sense of horror of going to prison. And I still had no idea for what, other than combining functional and cosmetic surgeries, which was standard operating procedure for plastic surgeons. Obviously the billing was the rub, but it wasn't my billing.

"It's your surgery. Without that surgery there couldn't have been any billing," Carmen said. "You were paid, and now they want you to pay for being paid. Right or wrong, they're going to indict you. And then it's up to me," he said, smacking his lips like a hungry lion at the prospect of a meal.

Karen sat there weeping. She still was in mourning for the cat, and this put her over the edge. "But you promised…" she sputtered.

"I didn't promise anything!" Larry said indignantly. "The only thing I promise is the best defense money can buy."

"But it wasn't supposed to come to this, to arrest and trial and…" Karen continued sputtering.

"Well, it has," Larry said. "And that's the way it is."

I felt like a deer caught in the headlights. A disaster was in progress, and somehow I couldn't stop it. It just got worse and worse. The best defense money can buy was going to cost me at least $500,000, Carmen gleefully calculated. It was indeed cheaper than my house, but not by much. I asked if it was too late to go back and take the immunity deal. Carmen rolled his eyes impatiently.

"This is law," he said. "There are no games here."

It seemed like a huge and cruel game to me. The whole trial process could take another two years, Carmen told us. There would be lots of hearings and investigations and discovery, and then a trial, possibly a long one. Look what I was getting for $500,000. He tried to make it seem like a bargain. And what if everything went wrong? Carmen didn't want to answer that. He implied that for $500,000 nothing would go wrong. Still, Karen pressed him, what are sentences for criminal fraud? "Five, ten years," he said gravely. "Five hundred thousand dollars is cheap compared to that."

Kiss my practice good-bye, I thought, as I would spend what was left of my life in the snares of the legal system. Kiss my life good-bye, as well, as I thought of what the stress of this so-called due process was going to do to my immune system. The cancer monster would see a crack in the wall and come roaring right in. Karen and I staggered out of the castle, betrayed, shocked, appalled at what lay ahead. This is what $85,000 had gotten me: a two-year stay of execution and the new opportunity to spend another two more years and $500,000. Why, oh, why didn't I just go to that first grand jury summons by myself, speak my piece, and get it over with?

There's an expression that a lawyer who represents himself has a fool for a client; the way I looked at it, Larry Carmen had one as well. I was that fool. Carmen had turned down a deal that would have been a real deal for me, but not for him; total immunity would have ended his billing spree. The government, he admitted, had told him they thought I was a "nice guy," a nice guy sick with cancer, but that didn't matter to Carmen. Nice guys finished last in his book, and in his ledger. If I had taken the transactional immunity deal, there would have been no further need for Larry Carmen. It was a matter of zero versus $500,000.

My arraignment took place a week later at the Federal Building in Westwood, high above the post office where I had gone countless times on innocent mailing missions. The FBI occupied two floors above.

That's where I reported with Rich Feig. Carmen had a court appearance that morning and couldn't make it. Rich could handle this by himself. I tried to rationalize that I was saving a few thousand in hourly fees, but I still felt a little abandoned. Karen, at my insistence, stayed home. I didn't want her to see her husband go through the legal process. I lied and said it would just be a lot of boring red tape, insisting that she take care of the office and allay any suspicions as to why I was absent. If having cancer could decimate a practice, being indicted for a felony could destroy it altogether.

What followed was probably the most humiliating day of my life. There were mug shots, fingerprints, and endless forms. My picture was taken with the usual set of numbers under the photo. They printed each of my fingers, my palms, my elbows, until I was covered in black ink that no Handi Wipe could get off. It remained indelible for weeks afterward, a black badge of my new criminality. The FBI agents who kicked this party off two years ago, Clint and Sigrid, were there, as was the U.S. Attorney in charge of my case, a Robert Redford look-alike with the unlikely name of Leander Peres.

The government team had an entire table stacked with evidence against me. But the charges, which I learned for the first time, were rather paltry. I was being charged with four counts of mail fraud. They were calling it mail fraud, because the center had sent its bills to the insurance companies by post, which therefore made it a federal offense. Had they delivered it by hand, I wondered whether I would have been here at all. The gravamen of the case was the same old FBI song, that there had been a commingling of functional and cosmetic surgeries, for which I had earned a grand total of less than $12,000 out of a gross revenue to the Beverwil Surgery Center of $40,000 (for anesthesiology, the use of the operating room, nurses, etc.) Yet for my $12,000 Carmen was expecting me to spend $500,000 to buy my freedom. My brilliant career was about to go up in smoke over $12,000 in disputed charges. It seemed all wrong, as did everything about the whole situation.

Rich Feig remained mostly silent during my processing ordeal. There were few words of support, of encouragement, of hope. I imagined he didn't want the FBI to hear anything. Every chair, every wall, every urinal in the Federal Building was surely tapped. Afterward, he took me down into the basement Federal Building for a cup of coffee. The cafeteria was cold and windowless, a preview of the prison that might lay ahead. The Yale man began talking of what came next, a court arraignment, then the first appearance, in which I would make my not guilty plea, then…

"I'm going to plead guilty," I said impulsively, out of nowhere, out of my mind.

Feig just stared at me as if I were as crazy as I sounded. The normally stone-faced young lawyer slowly cracked a smile, then emitted a small chuckle.

"I'm not going to plead not guilty," I said. "Enough is enough."

"But you're not guilty," Feig said. "Doctor, this takes time. Sure, it's nasty and long and ugly and unfair as hell, but that's the system. That's the game." Both the emperor and his Yale man always referred to this torture as a game. Some game. Fun.

"Game's over for me," I said. "I can't take this anymore."

"Can you take prison?" Feig asked me.

I really didn't think I would go to prison. However, I had read about poor people going to prison for life for stealing a slice of pizza in those "three strikes" cases. But down there in that fluorescent basement,

I just snapped. I decided the truth would set me free. I would plead guilty, even if I wasn't, even if Dexter had done the billing that had sealed my fate. If cancer was no excuse for this, then I was wrong, and I would admit it. I thought I had a pretty good alibi: impending death. After all, people could kill trespassers in their homes in self-defense, so can't a man with cancer delegate clerical work to someone else? But if that wasn't good enough, so be it.

I was definitely guilty of bad judgment, of putting my faith in false idols. What Dexter Farnham and Larry Carmen had in common was greed, greed that trumped their talent, greed that may have been endemic in the white-collar superstar class in Beverly Hills. I was guilty of not shedding my Bronx-based inferiority complex. I had to stop deferring to these "great men" who turned out to be nothing more than deposit-only cash machines. So let the chips fall where they may, I decided spontaneously. Guilty. I would plead guilty, and atone for my psychology. I was proud to be an American. How cruel and hard could the government, my government, be to me? That was my thinking, muddled as it surely was, after a morning of black ink upstairs.

"Let's plead guilty and work out a deal," I said to Feig.

"Let's?" He said that one word and let it hang, looking at me as if I were truly insane.

"Yeah," I said. "Let's. I want to plead guilty and get this over with. I can't put my poor wife through two years of this. So what do we do?"

"We?" Feig seemed to have a problem, a big problem, with first person plural.

"We. You're my lawyers, aren't you?"

"Not at all. The Carmen firm doesn't do guilty pleas. We're defense lawyers," the Yale man said with pride and with an arrogant antagonism meant to shut me up and get me to write the $500,000 check. How dare this stupid client question the emperor?

"You mean you won't represent me if I want to plead guilty?" I asked. "You won't handle that?"

"We don't represent losers, Dr. Reiter. We're winners. We're here to fight and win."

"I can't fight anymore."

"Then we can't help you. Don't be foolish, Dr. Reiter. We have two weeks before the arraignment. Go home, get some sleep. You'll feel better…"

"I really want to plead guilty. That's it. I'm dead serious. I want to plead guilty. I really want this over."

Feig sat for about three minutes, just looking at me. Then he stood up. "Then I'm afraid we can't help you anymore. Good-bye, Doctor."

I was appalled. I stood up, too. "Wait a minute. I've paid you $85,000, and you're walking out on me?"

"No, Doctor. You're walking out on us. You're walking out on your own case. The Carmen firm doesn't do guilty."

"Then who does?" I asked. "You can't leave me high and dry."

"You're doing it to yourself."

"It's my life. This is what I want to do."

"There are a lot of criminal lawyers out there. Good luck," he said, turning his back on me and walking out of my life. I was all alone, abandoned, at the mercy of a building and a system that seemed to have no mercy. Yet, somehow, someway, I felt empowered. I felt better, cleaner. I was my own man, not Dexter's man, not Carmen's man. It was good to have Larry Carmen out of my life. The emperor had been deposed. I was taking the law, LA Law, into my own hands.

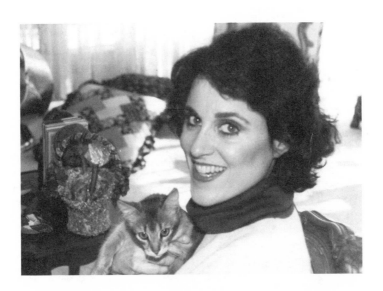

Karen with Wojge (above) and Mr. Tinker (below)

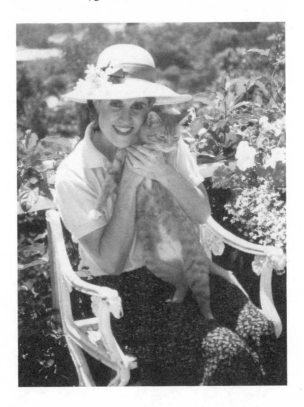

Chapter Eight

ANNUS HORRIBILIS
(A VERY BAD YEAR)

Karen was horrified that I had cut myself loose from the top criminal lawyer in the city. She blamed my behavior on the awful cancer; I blamed it on the awful lawyer. In any case, the order of the day was to find a new awful lawyer. I was convinced the adjective went with the profession, certainly as far as criminal law was concerned. Nevertheless, as an awful lawyer might say, it was a presumption that I hoped could be rebutted.. Maybe there was a great guy out there, but finding him in a matter of days seemed highly unlikely.

Again, we turned to Lee, who also couldn't believe my meshuggeh action. How could I have blown off the emperor of crime? I didn't even try to defend myself. Lee, to his credit and tolerance, came up with another good idea. He had a friend with the remarkable name of Hyman Law who was a distinguished California Circuit Court judge. When Hy's wife had developed breast cancer ten years before, Lee had had me speak to him. His wife had survived, and Hy felt I had been of great aid and comfort to him. He owed me one, Lee said, and Lee rang him to call in the chit.

Hy couldn't have been kinder. Because he was highly judicious, I assumed he would be reluctant to make any negative comments about

191

his esteemed colleague Larry Carmen, yet he came right out and told me he was deeply disturbed about my situation. He didn't mince words; in his opinion Larry Carmen was greedy, self-serving, and egomaniacal. His actions were reprehensible, especially in light of my health and my limited role at the Beverwil Surgical Center. Hy recommended a new attorney, Terry Galway, who had just left a senior position in the U.S. Attorney's Office to go into private practice at the downtown firm of McGreevey and McGrath. Since Terry had been the boss of the guys who were now about to prosecute me, Hy thought he would be the ideal man to defend me. I hadn't seen so many Irish names since I had lived in the Bronx where nearby Fordham Road, which led to the Catholic university of the same name, had been something of a Little Dublin. I remembered the Irish had dominated the police force in New York as well as Tammany Hall politics. They weren't the same force here in the Golden West, but I hoped that some of their Blarney Stone luck would rub off on me.

Where Larry Carmen was all flash and cash, McGreevey and McGrath was all business. The firm was housed on several floors of a new and anonymous office tower in downtown Los Angeles. Because LA is so vast and so decentralized, people from Beverly Hills rarely go downtown, save for baseball games at Dodger Stadium or concerts at the Music Center. It was terra incognita to me, and quite scary. In the shadow of those high rises were colonies of the homeless, lots of pawn shops, and many unsavory characters stalking those otherwise empty streets. LA had been trying to develop downtown for decades, but Angelenos' attachment to private transportation prevented the critical pedestrian mass that makes other cities work. I certainly felt safer in my car downtown, and delighted that McGreevey and McGrath had a guarded subterranean garage. It crossed my mind that the panhandlers and drug dealers who lunged at my car at traffic lights were just the sort of society I would be consorting with if the government had its way. Here was hoping that Terry Galway would prevent that from happening.

I met Terry with his colleague, Tim Pool, whose father had played a janitor on a TV show I had watched as a kid. Somehow this made the team seem like "real" people, even though nothing could have been much less real than that TV janitor. Both Terry and Tim were in their forties and very jock-ish, a match for all those blond Redford types arrayed against me. Both had gone to Harvard Law School, after Georgetown and Notre Dame, respectively. The very goyishness of it all reminded me of the august firm Dewey, Cheatham and Howe, but my first instinct about my new defenders was that I liked them.

There was little small talk. They got right to the case, which was more serious than those $12,000 would have led me to believe. Terry had talked to his former colleagues at the U.S. Attorney's Office. They told him they thought I was a decent guy, and they were sympathetic that I was ill with cancer. However, they were also frankly pissed off that, for all their sympathy, I had turned down their immunity offer, and now they were out to get me. It was a fabulous offer, Terry noted, but he wasn't surprised that Larry Carmen turned it down.

"There's no money in immunity," Terry said with a laugh. "Larry hung you out to dry so he could pick your pockets. It's a shame because you didn't need to be here."

Thanks, Larry, I thought. But here I was, and I couldn't look back in anger, or else I might be looking out from prison bars. As absurd as that seemed, Terry and Tim, while minimizing the likelihood, underscored that prison was a distinct possibility. "You'd make a great example, Dr.

Reiter," Tim said. "A poster boy for white-collar crime. Beverly Hills plastic surgeon goes to Lompoc. I would have loved a case like this." Lompoc is a notorious federal prison near Santa Barbara.

"But wouldn't Dexter Farnham make a better poster boy?" I asked. "He's the famous one."

"Hey, they'd like to make the two of you cellmates," Tim said. We all laughed, very, very uneasily. Tim told me he didn't believe billing issues were what the HIPPA law was intended "to get," but, as he also said, the law operated in mysterious ways. I had become frankly nervous about being a casualty of such mystery.

Terry and Tim told me that Dexter was trying to distance himself from the case, claiming he had no idea what I and the other doctors did, that he was only a landlord, renting out operating space to venal surgeons. And the billing? Dexter was blaming the surgeons for telling his secretaries what to bill, treating cosmetic as functional. He didn't have a clue. Just a lot of slick Beverly Hills doctors preying on poor Latinos. Terry told me how Dexter was portraying himself as the Latinos' best friend. He did, in fact, go on many relief missions to Central America after earthquakes and storms; he had even invited me to come with him. Karen had always wanted to go, to use her Spanish and love for things Hispanic, but I was too busy, and then I was too sick. Now Dexter, whose Beverwil Center made the vast majority of the money on these surgeries, was saying, "Blame Alvin." Dexter, I despaired, why hast thou forsaken me, and yourself?

Terry was low-key about his retainer. At $25,000, it was a twentieth of what Larry Carmen wanted, and I paid it gladly. It turned out that Tim Pool, the younger, cheaper partner, took on the entire responsibility of my case. But Tim was smart and sensitive and kind. In February 1999, Tim

194

stood beside me before Judge Martin Jones at the Federal Court House on Spring Street. Jones, according to Tim, was known as the Hangman because of his harsh sentences. He had been a POW in Vietnam. I suppose he knew all about incarceration. If it was good enough for him, it was good enough for the criminals who came before him. "Just our luck," Tim said ruefully. Before ascending to the bench, Jones had been a tax attorney in Beverly Hills, ostensibly aiding rich people avoid paying taxes. Now, in his new life, he had a particular animus against the white-collar types he used to find loopholes for. Tim filed several motions for a change of venue just to avoid the Hangman, but they failed. We couldn't get out of his dismal courtroom. I had moments in which I thought that perhaps I should fight after all. Why should I be railroaded into something I didn't knowingly do and that every other doctor did? Why shouldn't I stand up for my rights and those of my fellow doctors? Why, I wondered, didn't I have Charles Laughton in *Witness for the Prosecution* there to plead my case, to hang the Hangman? I wanted Laughton in his black robes, his powdered wig, his plummy upper-class British accent, "May it please the court, your honor," he would say. His words, his voice, his presence, his excellency—these would save me. But those were idle daydreams amidst a real nightmare. But I was too sick and tired to fight. "Guilty" was the path of least resistance, and, hopefully, not a path to disaster.

Karen sat in the first row of the gallery behind us, dressed in a lovely spring dress, the only thing bright and cheerful in the entire infernal proceeding. Although the courthouse was a grand edifice from the 1920s on the outside, inside it was as sterile as the '60s-era Federal Building in Westwood. There were dull, faded and peeling green walls, cold marble floors, and dim lighting. The ambience was prisonlike, though hopefully not a harbinger. Yet I got one step closer to those prison bars when I actually pleaded "guilty" to those four counts of mail fraud, all $12,000 worth. It seemed preposterous pleading guilty to something that was a common practice in the world of cosmetic surgery, especially in light of the overlay between cosmetic and functional components. But the government was obviously out to change that world, and here I was, caught in the crossfire of the slings and arrows of this most outrageous fortune. I had to look at it not as the outrage Karen thought it was, but rather as an absurd odyssey, an odyssey in justice, just as my lymphoma had been an odyssey in medicine. I did regret deeply having to force my poor wife along on this trip.

Little did I know that soon Karen would begin her own, infinitely more hellish journey, and I would have to go along for the worst ride of any lifetime. I must note here that I probably wouldn't have been alive at this point were it not for Karen. Her loving and wise support throughout my medical ordeal had given me something and someone to live for, a true reason to believe. She had made order out of chaos, and that order provided the framework for me to pursue my recovery and the continuation of my career. Karen loved order, and she loved beauty. Not only was she a beautiful person, but she created beauty all around her, in our garden, in our house, in our office.

Every weekend she would dress in an elegant Victorian outfit and serve a perfect high tea in our wonderful English garden. She turned me from a black thumb New Yorker into a plant wizard, the Luther Burbank of Bel Air. With a waterfall in the background, gurgling limestone fountains, and chirping birds, the teas were very soothing, and very escapist. We would be surrounded by a profusion of multicolored dahlias and English primrose, soft yellow hibiscus, fiery red canna, cascading geraniums, elegant roses. The food was delicious, especially scones with clotted cream that Karen would take one bite of and put aside. She had amazing self-control, which was an inspiration to me whenever I was about to lose mine, which was often. Because Karen had been a miserable fat teenager, she never wanted to be that miserable again, so she lived an exemplary, healthful life. Having flunked the Duke Rice Diet as a young woman, she had gone on to discover Weight Watchers, and it had become her religion, in some ways. Her embrace of Weight Watchers was unusual for an agnostic who deplored cults, but Weight Watchers worked for Karen, and therefore she worked for it, tirelessly and with the genuine passion of a true believer.

On its surface, Karen's love of Victoriana may have seemed a bit odd, if not pretentious, for a nice Jewish girl from the poorer side of Beverly Hills. Her enthusiasm embraced Agatha Christie, Jane Austen, Gilbert and Sullivan, the gardens of Gertrude Jekyll and Vita Sackville-West, Chelsea boots, the Lake District, the romance of the Raj—all of it. Victoriana was a counterbalance for the cultural wasteland of pop trends and television gimmicks and fading stars and money mania. She was desperate for a real culture, even if she had to travel to a different hemisphere and a different century to find it.

Karen's Anglophilia was genuine, as was her decision to go into the barrios and teach English to poor Latino immigrants. Hers wasn't a White Man's Burden English colonial missionary zeal; it was a true desire to bring order and beauty into the chaos of our lives. In the schools, she inspired students who had nothing to have dreams and make them come true. She had a wonderful gift for language, and in the classroom spoke fluent Castilian Spanish. In the garden she brought order to an unruly nature. She put up an old English sign in our garden and she lived by its words: "The kiss of the sun for pardon, the song of the birds for mirth, One is nearer God's heart in a garden than anywhere else on earth."

In our office, she helped patients understand their strengths and maximize their beauty, just as she had conquered her unruly appetites and become beautiful herself. She saw plastic surgery as an art as well as a science, and helped communicate my goals to the patients as well as help them articulate their own. She mastered human anatomy, surgical techniques, and the endless possibilities of surgical results as well as if she had completed a formal surgical training program in medical school. Her intelligence and kindness humanized the medical aspects of my practice, and made patients choose me over the countless other plastic surgeons in Beverly Hills fighting for the beauty business.

Karen was my Exhibit A, my trump card. She empathized with the patients in an uncanny, almost psychic way. She understood their fears, their fantasies, and their dreams, and she worked with me tirelessly to help make their dreams come true. Always inquisitive about everything, Karen had once applied for and won a position at the CIA in Washington. Fortunately for me, she turned it down. But I always amused myself by thinking about my wife in the CIA. Had she been there, world peace would have surely been upon us right now.

Karen had given me a real love life when I might have become one more playboy doctor. She gave me a family of cats when we couldn't have one of people. Above all, Karen's stability kept me from losing my mind, from succumbing to despair when I got sick from cancer, from wasting away from paranoia when I got into the crazy legal trouble, from dying of heartbreak and betrayal when my idols let me down, for convincing me to be my own idol.

This was a woman who loved and lived for order, who refused to let cancer, the bull in the china shop of our existence, upset the order of my life, and of our lives together. Above all, she lived for love, and I had the great good fortune of being the man she loved. Yet cancer was all around her, and not just in me. It had taken her handsome father, turning him from a Tyrone Power look-alike to a broken shell in short order. It had attacked her beautiful moviestar of a mother and her sister. Perhaps part of Karen's quest for order was to construct a fortress for herself when that malignant bull came her way, as she may have thought was inevitable, given her family history. She would never say it, because that would be bad luck, but she may have thought it, and she may have prepared for the worst. And then the worst happened.

It happened slowly, a stealth attack. I remember the date, May 17, a date that will live in infamy. I was back in court with Tim Pool before the Hangman for the first time since my guilty plea in February. We were making some sort of plea, for discovery, or whatever. I didn't realize that justice was so slow even when you were giving up. I thought I'd plead guilty, the lawyers would talk turkey with the judge, and I'd get it over with. But, not so. Because the Hangman was the Hangman, and there was the real chance I'd get prison time or some other cruel and unusual punishment, Tim was forced to proceed with all deliberation and caution, exercising every right I had, proving how clean I was and how dirty the others were, and basically dragging it out as long as possible, as if time would defuse the Hangman's wrath.

Karen went with me that morning, and that afternoon, when I went back to the office to try to maintain some sense of normalcy in my diminished practice, Karen went for her annual mammogram. This particular one was fraught, because Karen's mother's breast cancer had just begun to metastasize after nearly a decade of remission. Mimi, who was now 80, had had a double mastectomy in 1989; Karen's older sister had lost one breast in 1990 and the other in 1998. Gail was fine, but Mimi's cancer was spreading. Karen was deeply attached to her mother; the prospect of losing her was real now, and deeply upsetting to her. As if Karen didn't have enough to worry about, not only with my legal problems, but also with my own cancer. My six-year period, in which more than half of all patients with my kind of lymphoma would be dead, was approaching next year, and Karen and I were both highly aware of this D-day. So every event where something could possibly go wrong was a land mine of anxiety.

It was thus a great relief when Karen's mammogram came back normal. I wanted to take her out to celebrate, but she refused, not only on the principle *kinahurra*, but because she was feeling so sad about Mimi. Karen actually thought the mammogram was a mistake, that it had been read incorrectly. It was as if she didn't trust the good news, given that there had been such bad news all around us. I put on my rational doctor's hat and explained how mammograms worked and that she was fine, and that she should enjoy being fine. She put on her beautiful smile, but I suspected she was only trying to cheer me up.

Karen's grace period lasted about a week. She kept examining her breasts, looking for lumps, while I chided her for being neurotic. But on May 25, she got her "Eureka!" moment. "Look at this!" she announced, almost defiantly. Sure enough, she had found a tiny indentation below her left nipple and below that, an equally tiny lump. I felt it, and it did feel nodular, but Karen had always had fibrocystic breasts with many small benign lumps. If anything was wrong, the mammogram would have picked it up. Neither Mimi nor Gail had fibrocystic disease, as it was known.

Breast cancer wasn't a family curse, I tried to assure Karen. The little indentation was nothing. Give yourself a break, I begged her. But Mimi's cancer had super-sensitized her. And I wasn't a breast specialist, and, no, mammograms weren't perfectly foolproof. And Karen did take great pride in the sixth sense she had. Yet now she was using it against herself, and I hated seeing her so tortured. So for Karen's peace of mind, we decided to go to the best breast cancer specialist at Cedars, just to put the idea of a family curse to rest.

Carlton Starr was one of the nicest doctors I had ever met, a sixtyish, outdoorsy, world-class cancer surgeon without a trace of egomania that was otherwise endemic in the field. These guys were the true lifesavers, but Carlton was shy and modest. Going to him, I thought, was overkill in Karen's unlikely situation. But I had the connection, and I wanted to bring some serenity into a life I had taken so much from. So it was Carlton, once and for all, the highest authority, to lay this issue to rest. His office was as plain as he was. He took a great interest in what I was doing. Instead of the other recent events in my life, I talked of my lymphoma being in remission.

Then Carlton examined Karen. "It doesn't feel like anything. It certainly doesn't feel like cancer," he said. Still, just to cover all bases, he did a routine needle biopsy. Then he said, "I'll see you in six months." But what about the biopsy results, Karen pressed him. "I'll call with the results, if you want," Carlton said, implying there would be no need to call at all.

Two days later, we got a call at night at home from a deeply chagrinned Carlton Starr. "Karen, you've got cancer," he said sadly. I realized that Carlton had no choice but to give us this news on the phone. Had he said, "I need to see you in my office," we would have immediately known anyway. All I could think of when I heard the news was a billboard I had seen on the Sunset Strip years before promoting a gimmicky dating book. "The three cruelest words in the English language," the billboard trumpeted. "Let's Be Friends." That billboard was wrong. The three cruelest words in the English language were, "You've got cancer."

Karen didn't break down, didn't even cry, didn't even let me have it for doubting her mystical intuition. There were no "I told you so's." Just a quiet resolve to beat this awful disease. I was numbed by the news and by Karen's reaction.

The next day, we went back to see Carlton, and in the privacy of his office, we talked about what to do next. He outlined the next step, one he did not believe would have been necessary only a few days before. He planned a larger excisional biopsy, or lumpectomy, to remove as much of this tissue as possible and to include a rim of normal tissue for a margin of safety. Whether the margins were clear of cancer would be determined by the pathologist.

Carlton then examined Karen's breasts for any other obvious signs of cancer and found none. As I sat there, I remembered an old adage that has slipped out of our collective memories. Later I went to my library and looked it up. The AMA's first code of medical ethics, written in 1847, goes like this:

"The life of a sick person can be shortened not only by the acts, but also by the words or the manner of a physician. It is, therefore, a sacred duty to guard himself carefully in this respect, and to avoid all things which have a tendency to discourage the patient and to depress his spirits."

How this would come back to haunt us!

The surgery took place a few days later at Cedars-Sinai. I paced nervously in the waiting area, a role I was not accustomed to. When Carlton came out of the OR, he told me that the operation was successful. The next day Carlton, Karen, and I sat in his office to look at the big picture. Although Carlton's operation had removed Karen's cancer, he could not unconditionally guarantee that it would not return. Karen now "had cancer" and that was bad news, news that drastically affected Karen's view of a future already clouded by my own health and my legal issues.

Breaking bad news has to be one of the most difficult tasks that we doctors must perform. Carlton, with his reassuring manner, was more than up to this task. Karen had every reason to be as fragile as a rose in a winter storm, but she turned out be a rock of determination. She was so beautiful, so delicate, so vulnerable, even now in the middle of a maelstrom of a nightmare. A cancer diagnosis takes the words right out of you. But not my wife! Instead of cowering at cancer's fury, she stunned both Carlton and me by announcing that she was going to fight back, and fight back hard. She wanted to have a mastectomy. Not just a mastectomy of the breast that Carlton has just removed the lump from, but a double mastectomy.

Then Karen explained the method in what we at first saw as madness. This discovery of what seemed to be a tiny cancer in its earliest stage had put her on a kind of red alert. Remember the line that killed Barry Goldwater's Presidential campaign in 1964? "Extremism in the defense of liberty is no vice." That got him labeled as a right wing overreacting warmonger who would pull the nuclear trigger, though it probably would have served him well in our current patriotically security-conscious times. Well, Karen's position was that extremism in the defense against cancer was no vice, either, but rather a life-saving necessity. And she argued that position, not out of hysteria, and not with self-pity, but with an unassailable logic that the great jurist Oliver Wendell Holmes would have admired.

Not only did her mother and her sister have recurrent breast cancer, first in one breast, then, eight years later, in the other, but Karen told us that she had found out that her maternal grandmother had also died of it, as had numerous aunts and other relatives. I hadn't known this because Karen didn't like talking about it. Silence, she had hoped, would drive the cancer away, a cross of muteness to this malignant vampire. Even her virtuous Weight Watchers diet of fresh fish and green and yellow vegetables, which I always assumed was a function of vanity and control, was actually a bulwark against cancer. Now that all the bulwarks had failed, Karen was prepared to be as radical in defense of her life as she had been in her diet. "Take them off!" she insisted. Her sixth sense, which had never failed her, was telling her the wolf of cancer was at her door and the only way to repel it was to remove any sources of its nourishment.

Carlton was very conservative, and he didn't believe in losing a millimeter more of your body than you absolutely had to. "Take them off," Karen insisted. "I want to live."

Karen had read just about everything about breast cancer there was to read. This was anything but an uninformed decision. Both Carlton and I realized this. After about an hour of remonstration, we understood that this was no on-the-spot impulse but a choice that Karen had been rehearsing for her entire life, especially following her mother's and sister's cancers. Her whole life was watching her own tragedy unfold. Further compounding the loss was the beauty of Karen's breasts, perfect D-cups

204

that would have been the envy of every movie star in Hollywood. Karen was never vain about them, never wore flashy, revealing clothes, again, perhaps, because of the hubris factor, or because she knew that one day, this day, she was going to lose them.

I began thinking of everything I had learned about breast cancer in medical school, odds and ends like how the Swedish physician Carolus Linnaeus coined the term "mammalia" to distinguish animals with breasts from all other creatures. I did a lot of reading and rereading, believing that somehow knowledge was indeed power, the power I needed to help Karen fight the battle before her. I reflected on how the breast has played many roles other than as the source of life-sustaining milk for the young. Its symbolism is all-powerful, representing maternal fertility and abundance. It is everywhere in art and literature. And, as an object of eroticism, it is perhaps the most indelible feature of feminine allure.

I recalled how breast tumors were described by the Egyptians 3,000 years before Christ, that Indian writings dated to 2000 BC mention the treatment of tumorous growths with surgical removal, how the most famous Greek physician, Hippocrates, feared operating on breast cancer for fear of killing the patient far sooner than the cancer would if left alone. Another great Greek, Galen, had attributed breast cancer to a black bile in the body, which he called melancholia. That's how I felt now about Karen's prospective loss of this most powerful symbol of femininity. But Galen also valued life over vanity and, insisting on the importance of complete removal, urged doctors to be sure "to get it all," to make a wide incision "so as not to leave a single root." Then there was Saint Agatha, the patron saint of breast cancer, who had had her breasts amputated by a cruel and spurned Roman emperor in 200 AD as punishment for her Christian beliefs. I recalled a painting in which Agatha was visited in her dungeon cell by St. Peter and Jesus so they could heal her wounds. I said a prayer to her for Karen.

The end of the Middle Ages was marked by extremes. William Clowes (1560–1634), the physician to Queen Elizabeth I, advocated the "laying on of hands," and for a time the afflicted were touched in hopes of being healed. The discovery of the lymphatic system in 1622 had the effect of promoting the removal of enlarged lymph glands and, later, removal of the cancerous breast and chest muscles.

In the nineteenth century, the English breast surgeon Charles Moore observed, "In the performance of the operation, it is desirable to avoid not only cutting into the tumor, but also seeing it. No actually morbid texture should be exposed, lest the active microscopic elements in it be set free and lodged in the wound." He was warning that cutting into the tumor would spread its toxins into the body. It was a lesson that would haunt us a century later. The first radical mastectomy was done by William Halstead at Johns Hopkins in 1894, and the discovery of X-rays in 1895 by William Roentgen was of monumental importance in the treatment of breast cancer. Yet despite a century of progress and countless volumes of research and fortunes spent on the development of treatments, the disease remains one of our most dreaded scourges.

Plan A, the double mastectomy, went ahead as Karen wanted, though without Carlton. He had weeks of long-planned major surgeries ahead of him, and he had to coordinate his packed schedule with the packed schedule of the plastic reconstructive surgeon, who would give Karen new breasts. Karen had a deep sense of urgency and simply couldn't wait. And Carlton empathetically urged her to follow her instincts.

So we chose the man who had done Gail's mastectomy, another superstar, Armando Latini, at St. John's Hospital, a dashing, Ferrari-driving Milanese cancer surgeon who had originally been lured to America by UCLA, one of the country's best-funded university hospitals (with movie mogul money, such as the multimillion dollar pledges from the producer David Geffen and talent agent Mike Ovitz). Latini was a pioneer in sentinel node surgery, a procedure in which only the lymph nodes to which cancer has spread are removed. Not wanting to make the same mistake I had with Ted Kram, we also enlisted a top breast reconstruction surgeon, a courtly Southern gentleman, Dabney Lee, to begin the implant process simultaneous with the mastectomy, scheduled for early July.

We tried to spend the month of June getting psychologically ready for our impending loss, trying to enjoy our home, our garden, our cats, each other, and our patients. I guess we lived in denial of what was about to happen, but we were happy. Alas, Mimi was getting worse and weaker, and we spent a lot of time with her, keeping the secret of Karen's impending surgery to ourselves.

One secret that couldn't be kept under wraps was the muddle with the FBI. In the middle of June, the U.S. Attorney's Office issued a press release that "two prominent Beverly Hills plastic surgeons" had been indicted for multiple counts of mail fraud and faced potential prison terms of decades. The government had been out to make an example. It was just Dexter and me. I never thought I'd make the newspapers, except maybe for developing a cure for cancer, but not this. I remember reading about the edict of high society women to their children about having their names in the newspaper only three times in their lives: birth, marriage, and death. How would those dowagers feel about billing fraud? The release, short but fatal, hit the *LA Times*, the *Beverly Hills Courier*, and the *Valley News*, all well-read papers in the LA area.

My practice seemed to dry up overnight. No one called even to offer support. They just stopped calling. Crime makes people in Beverly Hills more uncomfortable than anything except poverty. Not that crime doesn't occur. Many of Beverly Hills' greatest estates and greatest fortunes were built on crime. Bugsy Siegel had been a pillar of Rodeo Drive society. Meyer Lansky was the toast of the town. Joe Kennedy, in his bootlegger days, held court there and owned a studio, RKO. David Begelman was rewarded for his Columbia Pictures frauds by being made the head of MGM. Producer and studio chief Robert Evans was busted for cocaine running, and ended up making more and more films. But movie people are held to a far different standard than doctors. Movie people are supposed to be naughty. Doctors aren't. It wasn't crime per se that was a sin. It was getting caught. That branded you as a loser, and nobody in this heavenly hamlet of winners wanted anything to do with a loser.

That awful press release upset Karen as much as her cancer did. She had been so proud of me, the great surgeon. Now it was her husband, the criminal. Now I felt guilty about having pleaded guilty. I hadn't ever considered that there would be any publicity about this, that my name would get into the papers. I wasn't what one would call a strategic thinker about such matters. Other plastic surgeons, the ones who were advertising all over the country and the world, were also hiring public relations firms. I suppose they would have warned me about this; they would have told me that Larry Carmen was cheap, cheap at any price, even at $500,000. But Larry Carmen never warned me about the bad publicity, and I was too naïve to anticipate the ways of the media-obsessed world.

I began having second, third, and fourth thoughts about not going to the mat over this case, even though I still thought of it as a Kafkaesque parking ticket that had gone out of control. But I had made my decision, and regret was a wasted emotion. Besides, with Karen to worry about, I didn't have too much time for remorse about myself. The one thing that cheered me up was hearing a local oldies station play the Rolling Stones' song, "Yesterday's Papers." The refrain, "Who wants yesterday's papers?...Nobody in the world," reminded me that peoples' memories were short, and that this, too, would pass. As long as the Hangman didn't send me to prison. Given the weirdness of my life, nothing was impossible or too preposterous.

In early July, Karen had her bilateral mastectomy. She had to tell Mimi because, just in case, she didn't want to leave the world without having said good-bye to the woman she loved more than anyone else. Mimi, who had gone through this herself and was going through it again now, was amazingly strong and reassuring, given her age and declining situation. She had given Karen her beauty and her grace, and she showed it all once again, grace under pressure.

Karen was fortified by Mimi's love and unconditional support, her unwillingness to play Jewish mother and tell her daughter not to cut her breasts off. Karen was highly intelligent and informed, and if that's what she wanted, so be it. And so it was. The operation went perfectly. Her breasts were removed, as were all the potentially involved lymph glands leading from the breasts into the armpits. The sad irony here was that the surgeons found absolutely no trace of cancer whatsoever. Carlton Starr had indeed gotten it all in the excisional biopsy. But Karen didn't look back in anger, regret, or self-loathing for overreacting. She couldn't stand a life worrying about cancer. Now she wouldn't have to.

Not that there wasn't anything else to worry about. The goal was to get Karen's life and looks back to normal as soon as possible. To the latter end, balloons were placed in the former breast tissue area. Over the next several months, these balloons were to be infused on a regular basis with salt water to expand the skin and create a pocket in which to eventually insert silicone implants. In due time, nipples would also be created for these newly formed breasts, a true miracle of modern reconstructive surgery.

A week after Karen's mastectomy, just as we were nearly (Jewish superstition prevented irrational exuberance) congratulating ourselves on how smoothly things were going, complications—those damn complications—suddenly arose. Karen noticed that one breast area was more swollen than the other. I examined her and concurred. I didn't want to alarm her, but I was worried that she might have a hematoma, bleeding into the surgical cavity. This was where the blood was accumulating in Karen. Maybe it was part of the post-surgical process, maybe it had clotted and was healing, but maybe it was expanding. I called the surgeon.

Alas, Armando Latini had left for Europe to lecture. So I called the reconstructive surgeon, Dabney Lee, whose secretary said he was not available either. When pressed, she admitted that he was in town, but hosting his mother and sisters, who were in from Mississippi. I pressed the secretary, who patched through Dr. Lee whose picturesque drawl reminded me of Robert E. Lee. He had to fetch his kin from the airport, but he could meet us at his office at Cedars in four hours, he said. I put Karen in bed to rest, carefully watching (but not letting her notice how closely) to make sure that the area wasn't swelling any further, which would have been indicative of a serious hemorrhage.

Lee's practice was exclusively cancer reconstruction, so his office was in the Cedars Cancer Center, in the basement of the hospital near where I had gone for my scans. The walls were lined with cheerful, bucolic paintings, but I knew it was one big act of denial, a big lie, the evidence against it being all the gaunt, bald, yellow, waxen, ashen patients waiting and hoping against hope. These were people, like myself, with dates over their heads: dates until progression of the cancer from its always-temporary remission, dates of median survival time, dates of rendezvous with destiny. These dates were invariably in months, rarely in years. Our times were short, our horizons sharply limited, our hopes fenced in. We were all terminal, of course, but I didn't like to be reminded of it, and I wished Lee's office were in a more sanguine spot, like Roxbury Drive. The Cedars basement was as quiet as a cemetery.

Karen waited for a long time in a chair in the waiting room, as quiet as everyone else there. She was frail, and, to my eye, getting paler by the minute. I worried silently that she might be bleeding to death. Karen, by her very serenity, prevented me from going ballistic. She would put on a smile and hold my hand, as if I were the one in need. Finally, Dr. Lee came out to get us and led us into one of the examining rooms. He was dressed in casual clothes, no white doctor's coat. He was obviously planning to take the day off and had come in for us, for which we thanked him profusely.

After examining Karen and taking all her vital signs, Dr. Lee gave me the impression, albeit in a charming Southern way, that we were wasting his time. "It's normal postoperative swelling," he said. "Completely normal." Dr. Lee theorized that her body was having a slight reaction to the "expander," or plastic balloon in her chest wall. He suggested that she return home and rest. It was the old take-two-aspirin-and-call-me-in-the-morning response. I could see Lee was in a hurry to get out of there and back to his family. I still sensed something was terribly wrong, but since I had pleaded guilty, and especially since my troubles had become public fodder, my self-esteem had sunk to less than zero. Who was I, a soon-to-be-convicted felon, to challenge the authority of this pillar of rectitude? Then I looked at Karen, and I saw how unconvinced she was too by Dr. Lee's assurances.

"You know, Dr. Lee," I said. (Pre-guilty plea I would have called him Dabney and treated him as an equal.) "I think it's acting more like a hematoma. From my observations since this morning, I'm afraid it could be expanding."

Dr. Lee gave me a long, quizzical look. Then he turned and walked out of the room. I thought that I had somehow offended him, and that he had stormed out in a pique. But Southern gentlemen didn't behave that way, even when they worked at Cedars. They stood up for their honor; they didn't walk out on it. Before Karen and I could figure out what was happening, Dr. Lee returned, now dressed in his white doctor's coat. In one change of clothes, he had gone from man to superman. He was holding a small syringe with a needle. "Let's see what's going on here," he said. Then he stuck the needle into the swollen cavity and drew out fresh, bright red blood. A look of total surprise overtook his face. "Good thinking, Doctor," he said to me. "It *is* a hematoma." My thirty-three years of medical training had paid off, and, for a brief shining moment, I had my old dignity back. More important, it turned out that I had saved Karen from bleeding to death.

Dr. Lee insisted that Karen remain in the hospital, for safety's sake. Like a little girl, she begged him to let her go home. She promised that she'd behave, stay in bed, not run around. But Lee had made one nearly fatal error; he wasn't about to make another. Besides, he had to bring her into the operating room to drain the bloody cavity and try to stop whatever was bleeding.

Even with the orders of one of Cedar's most distinguished surgeons, it took us ten hours before Dr. Lee could get an operating room for Karen. Maybe he took his family to Disneyland and then came back, but he seemed too concerned to have left her. The poor woman had to go through the endless admission drill, then wait for hours in a windowless broom-closet-sized room, without a bed to lie on—all this while possibly hemorrhaging to death. "We don't have any beds," the admitting nurse snapped at me. I wanted to snap back, "It's a hospital! What do you mean you don't have beds?" But I didn't.

I felt like Joseph and Mary, the no-room-at-the-inn syndrome, only here it was no bed at the inn. I wanted to call Dr. Lee but couldn't, as this was just before the advent of cell phones and our closet didn't have a line of its own. Karen stayed far calmer than I. I paced endlessly, imagining her going into shock from blood loss. I imagined a Code Blue. I imagined her dying just before we could get inside an OR. That's what ten hours in a broom closet can do to even the most measured of doctors. At my lowest, I blamed myself. Maybe it was just me. Everyone else got an OR.

At around 11 p.m., mercifully, before I lost my mind, Karen was finally wheeled into the OR. We were the last act of the night. I sat outside in the deserted waiting area. During the day, it was filled with families waiting for the doctors to come out with good news and glad tidings. I had done that many times during my own surgeries, for cancer reconstruction, trauma, or cosmetic procedures. It was a wonderful moment, the delivery of the all clear. I wondered whether I would ever be able to do it again, like in the good old days, which really should have been right now. I stared out at the twinkling lights of the mansions of Beverly Hills, at the graceful palms swaying in the moonlight, and wondered how this paradise on earth could have become such a living hell. Did every one of those mansions have a tragedy to hide, or was it just mine?

After about an hour, which seemed like five, Dr. Lee emerged. He gave me a smile. He thanked me again for being so sharp and vigilant. In his reassuring, stately tones, he told me how he had discovered the broken blood vessel that was filling up Karen's chest cavity. He had stopped the bleeding now, and he was sure that Karen would be fine. Of course he had been sure before as well. But I took the good news and thanked him profusely. I went into the recovery area, where Karen was lying pale and inert on a gurney. But she was alive, and I was glad. I kissed her good night.

Then I went home alone to an empty house, where our three cats, Doodle, Wojge, and Dexter purred at me and poured out their unconditional love, which I really needed. But they also looked around, in vain, for Karen, whom they clearly missed. They meowed for her. Their plaintive wails were eerie and sad; I felt the same way. I had to keep reminding myself that Karen was fine and would be back and all would be well now for her, for us, that the worst was over. I simply couldn't imagine a life without her.

When I picked Karen up the next day and brought her home, it was as if we had been separated for years, like we had both been off at war on two different fronts, and had been reunited against all odds. And we had been separated for only one night. Well, that was how glad I was to see her. The breast reconstruction project would now begin in earnest. "What some women will do to get silicone implants," I teased.

And she would laugh back. She never was mawkish, never looked back and felt sorry for herself. She was delighted to have her life, and to have me, almost as delighted as I was to have her.

In September I was back in court with more motions, more delays. I was assigned to be interviewed by a probation officer. Not that I was being given probation, but this was part of the endless procedure, to be vetted to make sure you had the right stuff to be on probation and not go directly to jail, do not pass go, do not collect two hundred dollars. In all honesty, Monopoly seemed just about as real as this thing called justice.

The probation officer, named Casper Trost, was a faceless bureaucrat with no sense of humor whatsoever. He came to see me at my house, which dumbfounded him. I don't know what he was expecting, perhaps a crack den, but it was clear that he had never been in such a place before. He was afraid to sit down, thinking he was in a museum. Once he did, he asked me a million questions, trying to fathom how I had descended into my life of crime. He was surprised to see both Karen and Mimi there. Did he think they were my gun molls? Mimi, whose cancer was advancing unabated, was spending a lot of time with us, so I could look after her personally.

When Tim Pool got me a copy of Trost's probation report, I noted his comments about my "extravagant furnishings" and "overindulged cats." He seemed to characterize me as a decadent Caligula. Did he really think that Fancy Feast cat food *was* a fancy feast? Did he think I took the cats to dinner at Spago, that I bought them cashmere sweaters on Rodeo Drive, that I was enrolling them in the Harvard-Westlake School for elite felines? The Hangman would surely make a fancy feast of this, come sentencing time, which the judge finally set for the coming December. Merry Christmas, Happy Hanukah, indeed.

Meanwhile, as Karen got better, Mimi got sicker. She had been blessed with a long remission since her own mastectomy in 1989, but now the devil was coming for his due. After that mastectomy, Mimi, I presume because of her age, was not given chemotherapy but placed on the drug Tamoxifen, which blocked the effect of estrogen, which Mimi had tested positive for in terms of feeding the cancer. The Tamoxifen had held the cancer at bay for a decade, but then in spring 1999, Mimi was finally placed on chemo, which did no good whatsoever.

The beginning of this end had come when Mimi began to notice a multiplicity of small bumps under the skin where her breasts had been. The lumps were enlarging rapidly, but seemed to be directly under the skin. Accordingly, we took her to a dermatologist in Beverly Hills, a Dr. Jonah Feinstein. I hadn't had much luck with dermatologists when I got my lymphoma rash, so I was willing to try someone new, and Feinstein was a name everyone seemed to be intoning as if it were a mantra. Like the first group of dermatologists who were stumped by my rash, Feinstein was doing a booming trade in skin peels and laser surgeries. He wasn't a surgeon like I was, but that was no impediment to a doctor's desire to aggrandize his practice.

Mimi was about four decades older than the next oldest patient in the office, or else Feinstein did such a great job that he truly turned back everyone's clock. Feinstein himself looked oddly youthful, the product of an obvious facelift, hair implants, and a tanning booth. He took a very cursory look at Mimi and pronounced that she had herpes zoster, or shingles. To me that was a preposterous diagnosis, because Mimi's bumps were not painful, as shingles are, nor did they follow the nerve route, which a nerve virus like shingles does. I wanted to ask him why he didn't think this was a herald of breast cancer, but again, in my current state, I held my counsel. Nor did I want to bring up the dreaded C word in front of Karen and her mother. Trying to be politic, I suggested a simple biopsy. He refused. He had a $3,000 laser candidate in the next room. Why waste time with an 80-year-old grandmother? A month later, when the bumps were even more widespread, Mimi went to her oncologist, who noted the bumps and sadly lowered his head. They were the prime harbinger of the return of her breast cancer. Again I was right, but what good was being right in this sad case?

By September, right after my last court appearance, Mimi had to be admitted to Cedars because her urine output had dropped ominously. This was the final curtain, and Mimi seemed uncharacteristically anxious and uncomfortable. Who wouldn't be? Her oncologist, who had given her the last decade and hence had no right to be second-guessed, prescribed a tranquilizer, Zoloft, which made Mimi wilder than a cocaine addict. I quickly discovered why when I checked the dosage. Zoloft needs to be started very slowly, then built up. Mimi's doctor had started her at full speed. Her dose was for someone thirty pounds heavier and forty years younger. Her doctor may have been a superb oncologist, but as a psychiatrist, who should be the one prescribing an anti-depressant like Zoloft, he stank.

I did my homework in the *Physicians' Desk Reference* and figured out the right dose, though the Nurse Ratchet-like administrator in charge didn't like the idea of me trying to interfere with the doctor's orders, even though the patient was clearly going out of her mind. Maybe the nurse had read about me in the paper. That's always what I thought whenever a fellow professional gave me the Rodney-Dangerfield-no-respect treatment. After a while, we did reach the oncologist, who, without a sign of self-abashment, changed the Zoloft prescription to my specifications. We gave her an old-fashioned Valium, and she calmed down immediately, and from then on was much better mentally, if not physically. This same doctor who had been credited for giving Mimi all those years was now ready to write her off. Once her kidneys are involved, it's all over, he told the family, and Gail and Lee readily concurred with him, much to Karen's distress. Knowing how much Karen wanted to keep her mother here on earth, I tried to ride to some sort of rescue by calling in the top urologist I knew, one of whose billionaire patients had set up a massive cancer foundation with this doctor at the helm. After some basic tests, as well as an ultrasound, he concluded that her cancer, while definitely back, had not spread to her kidneys at all, that Mimi was simply dehydrated. He ordered fluids and simple drinking water, lots of it, as much as Mimi could drink. And lo and behold, she urinated.

Mimi got another month at Cedars, a month she might not have had had her kidneys been allowed to shut down earlier. I couldn't help but think that with the right interventions, she might have gotten a few more months. But I wasn't about to precipitate a family feud at the deathbed of the matriarch. I did all I could, for I loved her, too. She was the only parent I had left, and losing her, and her unwavering support and good cheer, created a terrible void for me. Naturally for Karen, her mother's death was the saddest day of her life. Cancer had now claimed both her parents. It had me, and it had changed her forever.

Had there been any vestige of a relationship between me and Dexter Farnham, my guilty plea served to extinguish it. He saw it as a total betrayal, and I was now the enemy. I still had some surgeries to do at the Beverwil Center, but the staff and other doctors there barely spoke to me. I was the Judas of Beverwil. I did, however, have my own supporters, longtime employees that Dexter had fired in a purge to protect himself from their testimony against him. One woman, Betty Lazaro, who was in her seventies and had worked as Dexter's chief nurse for thirty years, called me after she was cut loose. No one could have been more loyal to Dexter. She would take all his emergency calls at night and weekends and instead of calling him for answers, she would pretend he was on the other line and handle the patients herself, always seeming to get it right. She was a kind of ventriloquist, simulating Dexter's reassuring voice in the background. She knew all of Dexter's secrets, some of which, in her outrage at being cut loose without a pension or other long-promised retirement benefits, she shared with me.

Insisting we meet late at night at a coffee shop in a neighborhood where no one would see us (she said Dexter had a gun collection, which I had no idea about, and could be violent), Betty told me of the secret safe in Dexter's office stuffed with millions of dollars, which she would give to money launderers in the middle of weekend nights or that Dexter himself would take with him on the private planes he flew to the Caribbean under the cover of those humanitarian relief missions. Dexter, she described, was obsessed with money. His hardscrabble Okie boyhood had given him a fierce desire to transcend his roots and, once he had succeeded in so doing, a pathological fear of being poor again.

Once the FBI investigation had started, Dexter had gotten his personal lawyer, a former office boy named Jacopo Lopez, whom Dexter had sent through college and law school and hence "owned," to destroy most crucial patient records. For this, he rewarded Jacopo with a red Ferrari. It was all eye-opening stuff, but I never had been one for office gossip, so I took it with a grain of salt.

Then Betty told me that Dexter and Jacopo had often discussed doctoring the remaining records to make me the fall guy for the FBI. She confirmed what I already knew, that Dexter had cut back my surgeries because he knew I wouldn't knowingly cheat the insurance companies, and that was so much less money he could make off me. I wasn't a "program" person, as were the other twelve-stepping doctors, as well as Dexter himself. That was the tie that bound. All he had on me was my cancer, and that was in remission, hence a much less binding tie. No, Dexter didn't trust me. He demanded absolute loyalty, and I wasn't giving it. I was expendable. I was also frame-able.

My last face-to-face conversation with Dexter was at the center not long after I had entered my guilty plea. Sigrid and her FBI colleagues were coming to the office on a discovery mission and Dexter was preparing the troops. "Be nice to Sigrid," he ordered people sarcastically. "She's our boss now." Yet when Sigrid arrived, I noticed how warm and charming Dexter was to her, how she fell under his powerful aura, how she entered his private office with her perpetual scowl and emerged an hour later grinning and glowing.

After the FBI had gone, Dexter and I ran into each other. "A house divided against itself cannot stand," were his words to me, quoting Abraham Lincoln. "I'm disappointed in you, Alvin. I thought you were a man."

"Whoso would be a man must be a nonconformist," I threw back at him. I don't know how Emerson popped into my mind. "I won't conform to a crooked system. Dexter, I guarantee I'm a lot more disappointed in you. Money! Come on. Don't you have enough money? Don't we all?"

"I gave you shelter, Alvin. I took you in, gave you shelter from the storm. I healed you. I made you."

"A convicted felon," I added to his sentence. "Yes, Dexter, you're a great doctor, but that makes your fall all the more pathetic. To waste your career…"

"Whose fall? Whose career?" He broke out into a fit of satanic laughter. "You're the one who's falling, Alvin. You're the one who'll have no career. I'm staying right here." He took one last look at me, shook his head in disbelief, and walked away.

In my rounds with Karen and with myself, I ran into a lot of doctors I knew. None of them ever referred to my legal situation or the scandal involving the center, though I was sure it had to have been a hot topic at Beverly Hills dinner parties. There was never a word of support, an, "I'm sorry about the mess you're in." Nothing. It wasn't that they were shunning me. They just didn't talk about it. Maybe it was too shocking, too scary, too possible that they might be next. Then, one day on Roxbury Drive, I ran into a respected old-time ENT doctor, Dennis Wyman, who had been a colleague of Henry Rubin, from whom my first boss, John Lipton, had bought his practice. Dennis, unlike any other doctor in Beverly Hills, was totally candid with me. "I hope you didn't give any evidence against Dexter," Dennis whispered to me amidst all the gorgeous women passing by en route to Gucci and Valentino on Rodeo Drive.

At first I thought Dennis was covering for Dexter, but it wasn't that at all. "He's totally connected," Dennis continued, in a whisper. And he wasn't referring to the medical societies or the people at Stanford and Mass General. "All that dirty money he takes to the Caymans. He's mobbed up. He'll have you killed. Don't push it, Alvin. For your own sake."

I took a deep breath and looked around at all the affluence, at the passing Bentleys, at all the plastic surgery, a lot of which had been done by Dexter and the guys at the center. Living in paradise had made me so naïve and trusting. I had been living for my surgery, my patients, my wife, my cats, my garden. Money laundering, Caymans, Mafia, murder, FBI, prison? I had no idea what evil lurked under the Southern California sun. Was my paradise a fool's paradise? None of this had ever occurred to me before. But it occurred to me now, and it chilled me to the bone.

Under the orders of Tim Pool, I had indeed been cooperating with Sigrid and company. He told me I had to, or else truly run the risk of incarceration. Cooperating would be my way of atoning for having turned down the immunity offer. Although I didn't know that much, I did my best to share what little I did know. I relayed my one big experience of billing fraud with the anesthesiologist Jeff Cooley, who had carefully plotted with Dexter, unbeknownst to me, forging my name on forms only to enrich himself and Dexter.

I later learned that Jeff, prior to working at the Beverwil Center, had endangered patients' lives at the other hospitals and surgery centers where he had worked by shooting himself up with narcotics at the same time he was anesthetizing his patients. He was giving them drugs that could kill them in minutes if not carefully monitored, and how careful can you be when you're on Demerol? Jeff was found out and briefly stripped of his license by the State Medical Board. It was brief because Jeff had friends in high places, friends like Dexter. And now at Beverwil, working directly with Dexter, Jeff was endangering lives again, not on drugs but on the NASDAQ. He would leave patients when they were fully asleep under general anesthesia and go and talk at length to his stockbroker. At the same time his stocks were doubling in value, Jeff was fraudulently tripling his billed hours at work for doing less than nothing.

Somehow Sigrid got incensed that I had even mentioned Jeff Cooley. "I do not want to hear about Dr. Cooley," she said, snarling at me. "Dr. Reiter, the case is here." She pointed to the center of our conference table at FBI headquarters in the Federal Building, where I went for these "confessionals." "And you are here," she said, pointing to the edge of the table. "But if you mention Dr. Cooley's name one more time, I will throw you right back in the case again." She banged her hand on the middle of the table. Tim Pool later told me that Jeff had gotten my immunity deal and was the government's chief witness. Small wonder Sigrid didn't want to hear a bad word about him. She couldn't afford to have her star witness sent to jail, where he so richly belonged.

Another time, when I was recounting my final conversation with Dexter, the day Sigrid had been in the office, she once again leapt down my throat, "Are you implying that I am sleeping with Dr. Farnham, Dr. Reiter?"

"Where did you get that?" I asked.

"That's a very dangerous thing for you to say, Dr. Reiter."

"But I didn't say any such thing."

"But I'm hearing that implication, Dr. Reiter. Is that what you think?" Sigrid got right in my face. Something had hit a nerve, and she had gone psycho. "How dare you think that?"

How dare you tell me what I can think, I wanted to say. Instead I said, "No ma'am. That's not what I think. I never said that. Never thought that." It was like dealing with the Gestapo. At one point Sigrid tried to turn me into one of her agents. She had been intrigued by my comments about the plastic surgeon Goran Porec, who seemed like a far more venal hustler and fraudmeister than Dexter Farnham. His fake clinics had preyed on new immigrants with promises of free

Hollywood beauty. Goran would spend five minutes making a few cuts in a patient's nose to make it appear that surgery had been done. Then he would bill the insurance companies for nonexistent procedures, while the anesthesiologists and the hospitals, all in on the scam, would profit mightily. Intrigued by these sordid revelations, Sigrid decreed that I should wear a wire, have lunch with Goran, and trap him into damaging admissions of his crimes.

I balked at being such a rat, but Tim Pool said I had no real choice. So I called Goran about coming to work in his new operating center, and he graciously agreed to see me. He may have been a crook, but he was a charming crook. That's how he got so many patients. The fitting of the wire in the men's room of the Federal Building was worthy of the Marx Brothers. Why they didn't hook me up in a private office, of which there were many, I'll never understand. After nearly electrocuting me on the wet floor, then strangling me with the wire, we found that the recorder did not work. It took an hour of fiddling with the machine before I made the brilliant discovery that there were no batteries in it. So the agents went looking for batteries, and in the whole giant skyscraper Federal Building, there wasn't a single battery that fit this recorder.

So we went to Thrifty Drugs to buy batteries, and finally they sent me on my way just in time to meet Goran at Spago. He only ate at star restaurants. He liked to put himself in the power spot where opportunity could knock, always looking to connect with a potential new rich client, or richer investor, to fund his immigrant clinics.

Unfortunately for the Feds, Goran was so busy table-hopping that we never got a real conversation going, and nothing juicy came out, other than an offer to use his OR for my surgery. I might have otherwise taken it, but going from Dexter to Goran would be going from bad to worse. So ended my career as a government informant.

Whatever Sigrid's psychological shortcomings, she somehow made her case. That fall, the great and perfect Dexter Farnham entered a guilty plea to about twenty counts of mail fraud in cases totaling about $850,000. The government had been alleging thousands of cases, in the many millions, so Dexter had obviously cut a deal, hopefully not at my expense. There was always the awful chance that the Hangman might want to send both of us off to be cellmates at Lompoc to be the poster boys of medical fraud. I had many visions of Dexter and me sharing a cell, a possibility underscored when the judge scheduled both of us to be sentenced on the same day in December.

That same month I went for my annual scans to see where my lymphoma was. Given the stresses and losses and bad luck of this awful year, I fully expected the cancer to have come back. But it hadn't, and I took some comfort in the fact that if I could survive 1999, I could survive anything. Except maybe prison and a cell with Dexter Farnham. Which was better, I wondered, being in remission in jail, or having cancer and being free?

I figured I would find out later that month. I went to the bleak courtroom with Karen and Tim Pool prepared to face Dexter Farnham for the first time in months. But Dexter Farnham wasn't there, and the Hangman was incensed. Sigrid stood up and approached the bench with the lead U.S. Attorney. "Dr. Farnham's on assignment for us, your honor. He's doing essential undercover work for us." Undercover work, I marveled. Sigrid spoke so highly of Dexter it seemed as if she and the U.S. Attorney were representing him, not prosecuting him. Dexter was so cunning and charismatic, he had put the Feds under his ether. I might have to sleep in that Lompoc cell all alone.

The judge wasn't at all pleased by Dexter's absence. Nor was he pleased with the case against me. It had taken him months to finally realize that my actual profit from my commingled charges was only $12,000, not the $40,000 the center grossed on them. "Twelve thousand dollars?" the Hangman roared at the U.S. Attorney. "You better come back with more against Dr. Reiter than that. I WANT MORE!" the judge shouted. "Get me MORE!"

The Hangman gave the government until February to come back to court with Dexter Farnham and with more crimes against the state by Alvin Reiter. I thus ended the worst year of my existence a free man—free of cancer, free of prison—yet both were looming ominously near. The year 2000 was approaching, a new century. That was the six-year point of my lymphoma, the year I had a solid greater than 50 percent chance of being dead. I could only guess what the odds of imprisonment would be. Still, Karen was alive and well, and that alone was cause for a bittersweet New Year's celebration with Gail and Lee, family for better or worse. We watched the ball descend over Times Square and waited anxiously for computers to crash all over the world, for missiles to be accidentally launched, for cities to shut down. The way 1999 had gone, I fully expected Armageddon, but nothing happened. So 1999, a year of dreadful bangs, ended with a whimper. Now all I had to dread was the new millennium.

Chapter Nine

TRIALS & TRIBULATIONS

It's amazing how quickly you can forget bad news when you get worse news. Between Karen's double mastectomy and my legal woes, I had nearly forgotten that I was supposed to be dead. Well, not exactly dead, but as per all the actuarial charts, my particular variety of non-Hodgkin's lymphoma gave me a greater than fifty-fifty shot of shuffling off this mortal coil in this first year of the new millennium. But the cancer had simply been placed in my inventory of concerns, a dead letter file of death, taxes, and other unpleasantries.

And then I got invited to a funeral. The deceased was a former patient of mine, a lovely man named Julio Sanchez, who had been the chief of security at one of Beverly Hills' grand hotels. Julio had some nonsurgical sinus problems that I was able to help him with. He also had another condition, as noted on his initial patient information form, that immediately piqued my curiosity: non-Hodgkins lymphoma. I guess misery loves company. But it wasn't a case of I'll show you mine if you show me yours. I feared if I told Julio, "Oh, I've got that, too," that he'd flee my office and tell everyone at the hotel and all Beverly Hills would know me as the doctor with cancer, and there would go my practice.

Instead, I played a medical variant of Twenty Questions with Julio, as I discreetly inquired about his NHL in connection with my physical examination of him. My pretext was trying to find any connection between his sinusitis and his NHL. If he saw through, or was confused by what I was doing, he was too much the gentleman to say so. Indeed, Julio had the exact variety I did, and he had discovered it at the same time I had. He had had the same nervous reaction to Fludarabine, which his doctor, like Herb, had not warned him about. He had the same violent reaction to the Leukeran. And he had the same anxiety attacks over being withheld his chemo when his white counts were too low. He and I, both the same age, had a lot in common. Over the years, I was pleased that Julio's NHL, like my own, had gone into remission after chemotherapy, and he seemed to be living a full and happy life. Somehow, I felt that my survival was linked to his. As long as Julio stayed alive, I thought, so would I. I hadn't seen Julio for several years, and I certainly didn't expect him to die before I saw him again.

When his son called to say how much his father had liked me and that the family would be honored by my presence at his funeral, my first reaction was sadness, but my second was panic. I wanted to ask what poor Julio had died from, because a certain answer might portend that poor Alvin might be next, but I was polite, and I wasn't about to be a ghoul at a time like this. Still, curiosity was killing me.

I went to the funeral without Karen. The last thing she needed was to go to a wake. She also didn't need to know the deeper ramifications of my attendance. My darkest fear of death was to leave Karen, vulnerable as she was now, having lost her mother and a key part of her womanhood, all alone in the world.

The funeral home where Julio's ceremony was to be held was very close to Dexter Farnham's Monterey Park clinic, the venue that had precipitated my looming potential demise as one of Beverly Hills' leading plastic surgeons. What an ironic situation, I thought on that long, ugly drive through the industrial wasteland of downtown Los Angeles, that the splendor of the California fantasy could be annihilated by the reality of trying to help the poor people of this richest state. Julio was one of these poor people, one who had made good in the Elysian Fields of Beverly Hills, but he had come home to die. But of what, I pondered, praying to myself it was a heart attack, a stroke, an accident, a spurned lover (he was a handsome Latino, after all), anything but NHL.

There were about thirty people at the chapel of the funeral home, all from the family. I'm sure I was the only doctor there. I felt special being included. I also felt as if I was attending my own funeral. It was something from *The Twilight Zone*. I had never met the son, but from the age of the person greeting the guests, I assumed that was he, and I was right. I told the son what a fine man his father was, and what a privilege it was for me to have treated him and gotten to know him. The son reiterated how much his father had thought of me. With each sentence the tension rose. I had to ask the question. But when? And how?

Finally it just popped out. How did Julio die? He was so young, so strong, so... "Cancer," the son said. At first I was relieved, thinking he meant some other cancer, prostate, stomach, anything. The son described how it had spread from one part of the body to another, without specifying the parts. "Not lymphoma," I somehow said, as if to reassure myself.

"Yes, it was lymphoma," the son said. "Non-Hodgkins lymphoma." He sounded just like a doctor. I almost expected him to add, "The small B-cell follicular indolent type, you know, just like the one you have, Dr. Reiter." But it wasn't necessary. I got the picture, and it was bleak. "He thought it had gone away," the son added, "and then it came back and ate him up alive." I thought that mine had gone away as well. Maybe life, after a certain point, wasn't meant to be enjoyed, I thought. I cried for Julio that night, and I think I may have shed a tear or two for myself as well.

A month later I was standing in another funeral home, the federal courthouse on Spring Street, waiting to face the Hangman, Judge Martin Jones, who was going to pronounce sentence upon me, and Dexter Farnham. I was there with Karen and Tim Pool, who did his best to assure me I would probably get probation and a fine, but he would never make any guarantees. "You never know until you know," Tim would say.

The whole ceremony of standing up and sitting down, the Hangman in his black robes, and all the polite "If it please the court" and the stilted legal language must have reminded my Anglophile wife of the trials we had sat in on at the Old Bailey, the famous ancient courthouse in London, but Tim was no Horace Rumpole and this was no novel. It was the nightmare of my life. Still, it seemed like the Star Chamber crossed with theatre of the absurd. All the Hangman needed was a white wig.

Alas, we were not first. We saw the Hangman dispose of some other cases. In every one, he sent the accused to prison, for years and years. He was mean and angry. If this was justice, it seemed like frontier justice. And then Judge Jones finally got to the King of the Wild Frontier himself, Dexter Farnham, who refused to lock eyes with me, seated as we were on opposite tiers of hard benches in the unadorned fluorescent courtroom.

Dexter's lawyer, the colleague of Larry Carmen, made a sleazily impassioned pitch to the judge that Dexter was a mere landlord, unaware of how the greedy doctors who used his facility were cleaning up on these poor gullible immigrants who'd do anything to look like the "real" Americans they saw on television. He portrayed Dexter as a modern saint, a Father Teresa who traveled the world saving the victims of earthquakes, hurricanes, fires, and other disasters. It sure sounded great. It made me sick, because it was true. I had worshipped Dexter for these good deeds, wanted to emulate him, would have gone on his mercy missions with him had I not gotten lymphoma and my low immunity might not have carried me through the third world. That the saint may have been laundering millions in offshore accounts during these flights of mercy was not alluded to.

Then Dexter stood up to speak for himself. He held himself like a gunslinger, his hands on his hips, as if ready to draw, and swaggered to the front of the courtroom, assuming he could put the Hangman under his spell. "Your honor," he said, in an arrogantly condescending tone, "I believe you are an intelligent man." He went on to talk about "my mission" in charity surgery around the world, a mission that could not be accomplished from a prison cell. He had lives to save. He talked of his born-again philosophy, his religion, his love of God. He sounded just like an evangelist Elmer Gantry, or maybe Marjoe. "We have a world to save, your honor," he said, as if talking to the Judge over a dinner table. "Work with me. Do your heart good."

Dexter Farnham was a great showman. But he had made a fatal flaw, which was his assumption that the Hangman had a heart. "Thank you, Mr. Farnham," the judge said. Not addressing the great doctor as "Doctor" was the handwriting on the wall. The judge then proceeded to sentence Dexter to four years in prison and a fine of more than a million dollars. The money was chicken feed compared to what Dexter had salted away. But four years were four years, and no money could buy that back.

I got a very clammy feeling. If Dexter could go to jail, after his silver-tongued oration, after his virtual seduction of the agent Sigrid, after his cunning lawyer had played every ace he could conjure up, then I could go to jail just as well. I looked at Karen. She looked worse, paler, more afraid, than when she'd gotten her breast cancer diagnosis. When the judge announced those four endless years, Dexter didn't even flinch. I'm sure I evinced far more pain than he did. The Hangman ordered him out of the courtroom. The bailiffs flanked him and took him away, his wife and team of lawyers following shell-shocked in his wake.

Now Karen, Tim, and I had the dismal courtroom all to ourselves. Just us, the Hangman, Sigrid, and the U.S. Attorney, Leander Peres, a seemingly nice boy who had somehow decided to play cops and robbers and had become a hard-assed lawman. I didn't know tough guys like that from Bronx Science. Now I wished I had.

At Tim's insistence, I had written out an entire speech of contrition and remorse. "Don't be afraid to humiliate yourself," he had insisted. "It beats jail." I must have used the word "sorry" three times in every sentence. I apologized for my entire life, for being a doctor, for being successful, for living in Beverly Hills, for living, period. But now I had cancer, my wife had cancer, her whole family was riddled with cancer. We were being punished big time for having done as well as we had, but still, I was sorry, sorry, sorry. It was the most shamelessly abject plea for forgiveness that had ever been penned. Tim had read it and loved it. I felt like a bad actor who deserved to be yanked offstage with the old vaudeville hook. This called for Laurence Olivier, but I was more like Soupy Sales.

After some last minute maneuvering between Tim Pool and Leander Peres, Judge Jones looked down from the bench at me, and began speaking to me. He called me "Mr. Reiter," not "Dr. Reiter," which I took as a bad sign. Then he began with a long discourse about how he knew that I had non-Hodgkin's lymphoma, but that "It wasn't so bad." I gasped. The Hangman went on to say that his mother also had NHL, and she went on to have a long and full life. The implication was that NHL was no bar to incarceration, and that I could have a long and full life in prison being brutalized by convicted murderers, rapists, and child molesters. "Good luck with your cancer, Mr. Reiter," the Hangman said in closing. Good luck at San Quentin or Lompoc. "Do you have anything to say before I sentence you?"

I surely did. I was outraged how the judge began playing doctor with me and my life. Non-Hodgkin's lymphoma is one of the most complicated of diseases. It was highly unlikely that the judge's mother had what I had. There were many, many variations, and given that I had just gone to the funeral of Julio, who did have exactly what I had, I may have been super-sensitized to the Hangman's dismissal of my condition. I stood before him, shaking a bit as I prepared to speak my piece about how glad I was that my mother and my father were not on this earth to witness the shame I had brought upon myself. I was about to apologize to my poor wife, who thought she had married a brilliant idealistic physician, and instead got a felon.

But none of that stuff ever came out of my mouth. Instead, I angrily crumpled up my sniveling speech and dropped the ball of papers on the floor. I didn't look back at Karen and Tim, but I'm sure they were horrified. They probably thought I had snapped, flipped out, and was going to blow my case. I had snapped. Just as I snapped and dumped Larry Carmen, I was about to dump the judge, or at least not suck up to him. I had this chance, a last chance, to be a man, my own man, and

I took it. I shot from the hip, impromptu, and decided to let the chips fall where they may.

"I'm sorry about your mother, your honor," I said in a calm, unwavering voice. My voice echoed through the dead silent courtroom. "But you see, your honor, I'm sorry in a way that I am a doctor who can read the textbooks. The type of lymphoma I have, and there are many types, is a small cell, follicular B-cell indolent Stage IV NHL, and by the sixth year, over half of us with this variety of NHL will die. So, your honor, I probably will not live longer than another year or two." When I said that, I really, truly believed it, and I'm certain my plaintive sincerity and bleak prospects rang through that unforgiving courtroom. The Hangman looked up at me. I had him now, man to man, not defendant to judge. I knew he was all ears. I knew he was paying rapt attention in that dead silence all around us. I didn't compare myself specifically to the judge's mother, but I knew that I had made the point that not all lymphomas are created equal.

I went on. "I'm truly sorry for what I did, but I was, in all honesty, not thinking of bookkeeping, but of survival. I felt fortunate to be able to continue my surgical practice in the face of this disease, and I'm sorry to have abdicated accounting responsibility for these surgeries to someone less than scrupulous. I have not been charged for any offenses involving my own private practice, only surgeries done on patients from Dr. Farnham's Monterey Park clinic, patients under his control. Even in the face of illness, I was able to keep my own house in order. And in this other house, I have been charged with only four instances of commingling of insurance charges, out of hundreds of surgeries I performed there. No, your honor, four wrongs don't make a right. But many people who have septorhinoplasties, or nose jobs, your honor, also have breathing problems. Many. Many. It's not all about appearances, and it is a gray area for all plastic surgeons. So all I can say is that I wish I had been more vigilant and that all I have done could be reversed. But it cannot. Thank you for your understanding." And I sat down next to Karen and Tim, both dazed and confused by my impromptu valedictory.

The Hangman was silent for what seemed like an eternity. Then he spoke. "Dr. Reiter," he said. Doctor, not Mister. With that split second of professional courtesy, respect, whatever, I knew I had salvaged what could have been the darkest day of my life. What's in a name? Everything! "I'm sorry for your health condition and I really wish the best for you. But I do have to punish you in some way." He took a long breath, and rolled the options around in his head for another eternity. "I'm going to impose a $30,000 fine, no restitution, and a three-year term of probation. Additionally, I am ordering a sixth-month term of in-house detention."

Judge Jones told the lawyers to work out the details with the probation officer, the one who had noted my "overindulged cats" in one report, but who also noted that my home was like a "hospice," with all three occupants, me, Karen, and Mimi, all afflicted with cancer. The Hangman left the bench. Karen was weeping with joy. She jumped up and gave me a huge kiss. Tim Pool hugged me. "You scared the hell out of me," he said, "but you were good, damn good. Great, actually. He gave you the absolute minimum. Thirty grand and probation was the bare bones, rock bottom, of what the sentencing guidelines mandated. He wanted to let you go, but he couldn't. You won the Hangman's heart. And I never thought he had one. "

I think I never really thought I would be going to jail. That would have been too absurd for what I had done. But far more absurd things happen every day. I was just too logical to believe it. Sweet are the uses of denial.

Not that I was home free. In fact, I was home, and anything but free. The next day after my sentencing, the probation officer arrived at my home to survey the house for the monitoring device. The probation officer was a by-the-book bureaucrat named Max Marks, who always seemed very nervous around me, as if he was going to catch my lymphoma or Karen's breast cancer. So eager was Max to get out of my house that he left the device there for me to have installed. I called a Westwood electronics shop where I had bought a television, and they sent over a nice Australian boy to install the monitor. He didn't flinch when I told him what it was. "I'm Aussie, mate. We're all convicts down there."

Once the monitor was set up, Max returned with my ankle bracelet, which was actually more like a ball and chain. It consisted of a rough leather strap, to which a heavy three-by-three inch black box was attached. This would monitor my whereabouts, to ensure I was adhering to the limits that the court had placed on my movements. If I were to leave the house, even to go out into the garden, the box would alert the control center, wherever it was, that I was out of range, and then some action, whatever it was, would presumably be taken against me. My "watch time" was from 7 p.m. to 7 a.m. The other half of the day, I could go to my office, grocery shopping, chemotherapy, or other vital errands, provided that I keep a diary outlining my movements at all time. Max tried to suggest that people were watching me at all times, so if I slipped off to a movie, a restaurant, or anything vaguely pleasurable, they would know I had been violating the terms of my parole and I would immediately be incarcerated. I'm sure it was all scare tactics.

Karen felt totally violated. She had just recently completed the arduous breast reconstruction process. She had undergone several minor operations, removing skin from her vaginal area to construct artificial nipples for her new breasts. She had been in the hospital three days at a time for these surgeries; it was a long ordeal, but to her it was worth it. We even went to a medical tattoo artist to inscribe aureole around these new nipples. I half expected a hipster type to be doing the tattoos, someone who would also give Karen a heart on her shoulder, but the guy was a dull medical type. The tattoos did at least add some levity to a generally grim process.

Karen desperately wanted her womanhood back, or at least some rough facsimile thereof. The new breasts were not like her real ones, as silicone breasts rarely are. They didn't have her natural teardrop shape. Still, I was amazed at how good they did look, and how soft they felt. Furthermore, they allowed Karen to fill out her dresses. Now she wanted to go out and live a little, to enjoy the life she had made this ultimate sacrifice to save. But we couldn't. From dusk to dawn, we were prisoners of our bedroom. It was cruel and unusual punishment for a lovely woman who had been punished enough by her family's cancer curse. There was a lot to be thankful for, but my confinement put a pall of sadness over our life.

Still, Karen made the most of having me at home. The bright side, she reminded me, was that I couldn't be called to the emergency room at ungodly hours. She'd make lovely teas and candlelit dinners, and she rented wonderful old films, romances, epics, and foreign treasures, to remind us of what a great life we would have once we were free to have it. If I had to be confined anywhere, my house was the best place I could possibly be.

To be in solitary with Karen was probably the sweetest punishment a man could ever have. Her face was not only strikingly gorgeous, it was lit from within. She simply glowed. Her beauty was timeless. All the anthropometric methods I had learned as a plastic surgeon couldn't have produced a better result than Karen. It was poetic justice of the best kind that this plastic surgeon had such a goddess for a wife. But I must stress that the real beauty was how the inside matched the outside. The ravages of Karen's cancer surgeries had not dimmed her allure in the slightest; in fact, her inner strength enhanced it. I think Karen's was a kind of divine strength, and it made me endlessly proud that she had chosen me and loved me and stood by me, through times that would try any wife's soul. Her soul was boundless, and I have to thank the courts for giving us that time together. She could always make me laugh, make me forget what was supposedly a penal exercise. What was a sentence was actually a gift. In sharing that time, we finally got to savor every room we had spent so much time decorating. As a busy surgeon, the house had been basically a place to sleep, and not for that many hours. And then it became the best prison on earth. Yet I still longed for my, our, freedom.

Karen had a tailor let down the cuffs of several of my suits to cover my ankle box. I then began going back to my little office and seeing patients, trying to stay behind my desk as much as possible and never kicking up my heels. When I would examine patients, I was more careful than usual not to stumble over them. Because of Karen's ordeal as well as my own, I hadn't followed up on my plan to seek new doctor referrals and new operating rooms to work in. Dexter's conviction, and my own, did get reported in a very minor blurb in the Metro section of the *Los Angeles Times*, but it seemed to have gotten lost among the bigger stories of the day, and nobody had mentioned it to me.

I was sure the government was disappointed it hadn't made a bigger splash than it had. Yes, Dexter was a big fish, but I suspect the Feds expected to net a whole school of big fish, and they just didn't get them. Many doctors were doing the same things Dexter did, billing-wise, but they seemed to keep better rapport with their patients, who wouldn't testify against them. These patients didn't want to bite the hand that had beautified them. Dexter and his East LA henchmen, on the other hand, were running too much of an anonymous assembly line, and some of these patients, mostly friends of the nurse Dexter had abused for her fatness, were convinced to rat him out. His arrogance finally came back to destroy him.

Even though I was locked in at night, I felt, ironically, that my conviction had set me free. There was no longer the black cloud of the FBI and the U.S. Attorney hanging over my head. I had gone into the federal lion's den and had come out with little more than a nasty, clunky anklet to show for it. In six months, my life would be back to normal, and I would start networking and rebuild the surgery practice that had given me such joy, my professional raison d'etre. I would take Karen on some wonderful trips around the world, to make up for what I had put her through, and to show her how much I loved her. Perhaps I would take her back to the lavender fields of Provence, or maybe the crystalline waters of Tahiti, where we had scuba dived among fish so exotic that they seemed to come from another galaxy, or maybe just to New York for a marathon shopping spree on Madison Avenue.

Whatever we did, my main goal was to make her as proud of me as she always had been; although, never in the midst of this legal quagmire did she ever express an ounce of doubt, a smidgen of shame. She said she knew a raw deal when she saw it, and that was all this was, just another dose of bad luck. We both vowed it was high time for our fortunes to get back on track, and we looked to the six months expiry of my home confinement that coming September as our red letter day, when our luck would change and happy days would be with us again.

Then one day, just as we were crossing off the days on our calendar, Karen began experiencing pain in her right shoulder, elbow, and wrist. So we went to Herb Bloomfield, my cancer doctor, who had become Karen's cancer doctor as well. I had been seeing Herb since 1994. In late 1997 I was placed in the "watch and wait" mode, standing by anxiously for the complete remission sign to change. But it never did, and gradually, with each yearly scan that was clear, my anxieties began to subside. I trusted Herb and was deeply grateful to him.

Karen had first seen Herb in October, 1999, after the surgeons Starr, Latini, and Lee had done their respective jobs. Karen, always more than prepared, presented Herb with an all-encompassing medical and surgical history, a detailed report on her current state of health, and, importantly, the unmistakable family history of breast cancer, the history that Karen did not want to see repeat itself. Some dynasties pass fortunes from generation to generation. Karen's passed breast cancer. In giving Herb this detailed history, we assumed he would then send for Karen's medical records, including operative and pathology notes, indispensable for his treatment of Karen, and we gave him full releases to obtain these files.

After a cursory physical exam, Herb ordered blood tests, including one for a tumor marker. This test, for the CA 15-3 tumor marker, measures certain cancer proteins, and, while not foolproof, it can serve as an early warning device. Karen's result was fifteen units, the normal range being from zero to thirty. Any numbers under thirty may represent measurable but normal proteins, not the breast cancer protein. Although tumor markers are not high in every person with cancer, higher than normal levels can help doctors diagnose and follow some types of cancer, specifically Karen's newly diagnosed breast cancer. We asked Herb, pestered him in fact, about any other tests Karen should take. He reassured us that while vigilance was necessary, no further tests were indicated at this time. I thought for a moment: if not this time, then what time, but I let it pass.

We got very specific with Herb, asking about how the cancer looked under the microscope, its growth potential, the significance of the small tumor size (about three-eighths of an inch), the fact that no other cancer was found in the breasts or in multiple lymph glands. We also found out that a protein cell membrane called HER2/neu, which can promote cancer growth, was absent in Karen's cancer, a good sign. All the above was very encouraging, giving rise to an excellent prognosis and probable cancer cure. Herb stated, in his dull actuarial tone, that Karen's mastectomy had virtually ruled out breast cancer as one of her life problems, eliminating her greatest of all fears. Or it ruled it out by a stated factor of 95 percent, which was as close to a guarantee as any doctor, especially a deadly pessimist like Herb, would give. But that 5 percent still nagged at her.

The one finding that did bother Karen was that her cancer was determined to have what is known as an estrogen-positive receptor. Karen knew there was an ominous connection between a positive receptor and breast cancer. To the uninitiated, estrogen is the highly potent female hormone produced by a woman's ovaries that causes breast tissue to grow. It prepares the body of adult women for pregnancy and promotes milk production. Where cancer is concerned, it has been found that estrogen itself does not cause cancer but it does accelerate the process of cell proliferation and can therefore increase the chance of mutation or encourage the growth of cancer cells once they appear. Estrogen can play tricks on the body with its own version of Dr. Jekyll and Mr. Hyde. This hormone, responsible for fertility, strong bones, and a woman's overall femininity, has also been found to play a major role in breast cancer.

It was first noted in 1836 by the famed English physician Sir Astley Cooper that breast cancer was hormone dependent because it tended to wax and wane according to a patient's menstrual cycle. By the end of the nineteenth century, it had become well recognized that the gonads influenced a variety of tissues. In 1889 it was first suggested that removal of the gonads or ovaries should be performed before operating for breast cancer in order to prevent it from spreading locally or to arrest a rapid growth. Also in the late nineteenth century, another legendary English surgeon, George Thomas Beatson, became convinced that the ovaries sent out bad "influences," and he performed the first therapeutic removal of the ovaries for treatment of advanced breast cancer in 1895. This produced a tumor regression, though not a cure. This all remained an inexact science until the discovery of estrogen in the 1930s and of estrogen receptors in the 1960s, which led to the concept of hormonal management with drugs known as estrogen receptor blockers, the most famous of which was Tamoxifen.

At our first meeting with Herb, I didn't realize the full significance of Karen's tumor being estrogen positive. But Karen did, and she immediately asked Herb if he should prescribe Tamoxifen for her. Tamoxifen, an estrogen receptor blocker, was by no means a new or experimental drug. It had been approved by the FDA in 1977 for treatment of all stages of breast cancer and, in 1998, was approved as a chemopreventative agent for women at high risk for developing breast cancer (which Karen clearly was, given her family history). Thus by 1999, when Karen first saw Herb, hormonal therapy had meant Tamoxifen for more than twenty years. In truth, Karen met all the criteria for being prescribed Tamoxifen except one: the oncologist's recommendation. Herb simply didn't believe it was indicated.

Karen's mother had gotten Tamoxifen, as had her sister. So why not Karen? Because Mimi had died (albeit at 80) of breast cancer and because Gail had gotten cancer in her other breast after eight years on Tamoxifen, Karen, who had researched everything, couldn't help but wonder about the wonder drug, which did carry with it increased risks of uterine cancer, blood clots, and cataracts. (The benefits of the drug were generally thought to be well worth these statistical risks.) Tamoxifen was also thought to begin to lose its efficacy after five years, which may have explained Gail's progression, but that, in my mind, was not an argument against Tamoxifen. Five years was five years. I was all for it. But Herb was our doctor-in-chief at this stage, and we sought his commandment on this subject. "In my condition and circumstances, would you use the Tamoxifen for your wife?" Karen asked him.

Herb wouldn't answer her. He put it to the Cedars Hematology Oncology Group, a panel of eight oncologists who review cancer patients. And the group came back split, fifty-fifty. So it was back to Herb, and Herb cast the deciding vote against Tamoxifen treatment. In retrospect, we should have sought even more opinions, but we decided we might have just been driving ourselves crazy. That's why it's so important to have a doctor you can trust. Which we thought we did. That's what all-knowing doctors like Herb are for, to make the tough calls. But these calls are supposedly based on sound medical and factual reasoning. I didn't want to believe that a decision against using a drug that seemed great to me, was a bad call. Great doctors, doctors like Herb, weren't supposed to make bad calls. This one came back to haunt us terribly.

In retrospect—a worthless endeavor unless others can learn from my mistakes—this wasn't the only questionable call that Herb would make. Another involved the use of scans. I had learned in my medical training that whenever you are diagnosed with any type of cancer, that cancer must be "staged," which means to determine if the cancer has spread beyond its original boundaries, in this case, Karen's left breast. Thus I was surprised that, in 1999, Herb didn't order a bone scan and a CT scan to look for any bone metastases, which are often asymptomatic in their early stages. "Early detection" is a catchphrase of the American Cancer society. But Herb was my doctor, and here I was, vibrant living proof of his competence, if not brilliance, so who was I to bite the hand that helped me live. If Herb said the tests were not in order, how could I not trust him? I expected my patients to trust me. Turnabout was the only fair play, and besides, Herb was a big man in oncology, a man whom everybody trusted. To distrust him would be tantamount to medical treason.

Which brings us back to the onset of Karen's bone pain, in May 2000. I hated to bring even the word cancer, or oncology, back into her life. What she had, if anything, was far more likely to be just about anything else. But cancer was Karen's *bête noir*, and she needed reassurance. So we went to Herb, who had been following Karen since the previous October with blood tests every three months (though no more tumor markers, which he felt weren't indicated). The blood tests had been fine. All I really wanted from Herb was some reassurance for Karen.

It was a mistake. Going to Herb for reassurance was like going to Stalin for compassion. Herb begged off the case. He said bone pain wasn't his area of expertise. He didn't give us one kind word, not even a casual "it's probably nothing." That wasn't his way. But Herb had kept me alive, or at least I had stayed alive on Herb's watch, so I gave him lots of credit and overlooked his sorely deficient bedside manner.

So onward through the medical ranks we went. Our next stop was Kevin Porter, the dedicated rheumatologist who had diagnosed my lymphoma. If it seems as if I was looking for trouble taking Karen to these cancer doctors, that was hardly the case. These were top doctors, my doctors, who had kept me alive. I felt I was putting Karen in the hands of winners, men who would find out what was ailing her, deal with it, and let us start making wonderful life plans for my soon-to-end home imprisonment. Kevin was like Sherlock Holmes. If Karen had anything, Kevin would be the one to find it. I prayed there wouldn't be anything serious, that I could present my beloved wife a clean bill of health, and that we could finally start living the good life she had made such sacrifices to have.

Kevin was thorough as always, doing blood tests and regular X-rays of Karen's wrists and shoulders. Nothing. But leaving no stone unturned, he wanted more, and so did Karen. It hurt that much, and I took her cries of agony seriously. She may have been a worrier, but she was not a complainer. I once cut out for Karen, in healthier days, a cartoon from the *New Yorker* that showed a tombstone with the inscription, "I Told You I Was Sick." I had no idea this would be the case here.

But the bone scan Kevin ordered, which he said was to rule out arthritis once and for all, opened a horrible new can of worms. It revealed a large, suspicious lesion on Karen's spine. The shoulders, elbows, and wrists were all normal, and Kevin concluded that whatever pain Karen was feeling was coming from this lesion. "Lesion" sounds nasty, but it can often be benign. That's what I prayed for as we waited for the results of the CT scan Kevin then ordered in that gloomy Cedars basement. Alas, it was the worst possible news. The spinal lesion was malignant. A further workup revealed three other lesions, discovered in Karen's liver. The diagnosis: metastatic breast cancer.

Metastatic breast cancer? Karen had undergone a total bilateral mastectomy and removal of her underarm lymph glands on each side. The pathological analysis revealed no evidence of cancer. But how could this be, I wondered, if Karen had no breasts to get cancer in, and the post-surgical pathological analysis of the breasts indicated zero cancer tissue in either breast or in the lymph glands, none whatsoever? All the cancer tissue had actually been removed in the excisional biopsy by Carlton Starr. I figured two things might have gone wrong. The first was that the breast surgery had actually been incomplete. The second was that the breast cancer had already begun to sew its evil seeds before Karen strategically had her breasts removed.

When Karen's small breast lump was found, the doctors didn't explore the rest of her body with a series of tests such as a bone scan and CT scan to determine if the cancer had spread. The most common area to which breast cancer spreads, or metastasizes, is the bone. I had asked Herb if scans needed to be done, and he had stated no, emphatically no. And when laconic, low-key Herb is emphatic, you listen. The breast lump, malignant as it was, he said, was no call for a full-body investigation.

I had always thought that early detection of cancer was the best defense the body has, as in colonoscopies, mammograms, chest X-rays, and beyond. This advice is strongly recommended by the American Cancer Society and the National Cancer Institute, among many cancer advocacy groups. Why not then with Karen? How easy it would have been to do an early scan. What was one more test? Yes, Herb was the great expert, but I began to wonder whether I should have been less respectful of authority, my personal *bête noir*, and more insistent about my increasingly nagging doubts. I hated beating up on myself; nevertheless, those questions of "might," "could," and "should" made it hard to sleep in the days following this awful diagnosis.

Karen was beyond devastated. She was beyond the beyond. She thought she had beaten cancer, and now cancer had beaten her. It had tricked her, and me, and all these big league doctors. She felt betrayed. She had suffered the horrible mastectomy, suffered the horrible breast reconstruction and its multiple mutilative operations, all for naught.

Armed with his dismal diagnosis, Kevin hit the cancer ball back into the court of Herb, the great oncologist who would be the field general of the new war that we were about to begin. I wanted the expert to answer the big questions. I was a plastic surgeon, not a cancer doctor. I had had cancer successes in the past, many of them, but they were all head and neck work. I wanted the best answers, answers Herb could give better than anyone. Big mistake again.

Around the time of all of Kevin's tests, late August, 2000, we went back to Herb's office. He quickly examined Karen and said very little, and not a single word of the slightest encouragement. He said he couldn't really say much until he had the results of all the tests. The radiologist at Cedars who had read the bone scan held out a smidgen of hope that it might not be cancer at all, but a benign bone lesion. We thus hung on to any scrap of brightness we could find.

Herb did order some blood tests, and for the first time since he had begun seeing Karen nearly a year before, he ordered a test for the CA15-3 tumor marker. A few days later I called, at Karen's urging, for the result of that test. It was 115. I was floored. It was only fifteen last October, normal, perfectly normal. Why didn't Herb repeat this test each time we saw him? We were there in January, April, June, and July. He had taken blood every time, but he hadn't tested for what we were worried about, cancer. Instead he checked Karen's levels of potassium, sodium, sugar—routine lab tests. We didn't care about diabetes, cholesterol, or anemia. We cared about cancer, and Herb was Doctor Cancer. Yet he obviously wasn't worried, not even in June when Karen first went in complaining of bone pain, a harbinger of metastatic bone cancer. I later learned that these markers were routinely tested every three months. Precious time may have been lost, time that could have been vital to Karen's well-being. But now it was too late.

Karen was truly desperate for the first time in her life. She sat there looking at all the bad results, the scans and the markers that sealed a grim fate, trying to make sense of it all, trying to find that ray of sunshine in all the gloom and doom. If anyone could find it, it was Karen. Yet she couldn't stop herself from recalling her own father's miserable death twelve years before of metastatic liver cancer that had begun in the pancreas.

Woman of science that she was, Karen reached out to the man of science for some kind of life raft of hope. "Am I dying?" she asked Herb directly by phone. I cringed when I heard the question. I knew she was asking the wrong guy. The same doctor who had given her a 95 percent chance to be breast cancer free for the rest of a normal life now said, in a voice more flat than his normal flat monotone, "There is no cure for you." Those were the six cruelest words I've ever heard. I was destroyed; Karen, already reeling from what was going on, was beyond stunned.

Because the focus of my work had changed over the years from head and neck surgery to primarily plastic surgery, my scope and view of breaking bad news had changed as well. I didn't have to talk cancer. I might have to deal with a patient who was less than happy about her nose. It wasn't life and death. But I did know that Herb had just violated almost every bit of protocol on the subject I had ever learned.

The acronym for doctors is SPIKE: S for setting, P for perception, I for Information, K for Knowledge, and E for Empathy. Well, Herb got it all wrong. Wrong! It didn't matter that Karen had called him. All he had to do was invite us to his office. The setting should have been a quiet, private place, and we should all have been seated, to show us he had had time to explore all ramifications of the grim tidings. He should have found out all Karen knew about her situation, to understand her perception. He should have tried to find out how much information Karen wanted to know about her condition. None of this was ever discussed. He should have decided on an agenda: from diagnosis to treatment, including the prognosis and support system: knowledge of the plan of attack. Herb had to know this. But he simply didn't operate in the psychology realm, which was the last ingredient: empathy. Empathy? Herb? You gotta be kidding.

This humanistic skill wasn't taught in medical school, but Herb certainly had the experience and opportunity as an oncologist to communicate bad news to patients and family. Time spent honing this ability to communicate sad tidings would have had far-reaching benefits to all the people Herb treated. But it was too late for Herb; I prayed it wouldn't be too late for Karen. Forget SPIKE. SURVIVAL was the only word that mattered now.

Frankly, neither of us could remember the rest of the conversation. So much for our round-the-world trips. Now it would be round the Cedars basement. I took Karen for an outpatient liver biopsy at Cedars. I felt awful that she was thrust back into more surgery, like a guinea pig, but she was a great sport about it. It was the price of wanting to live, she said, and she vowed to endure whatever it took.

I had done some quick research and was floored to learn that someone Karen's age, fifty-five, with metastatic breast cancer had, statistically, three years to live. I took some heart from the fact that Karen's mother had had metastatic breast cancer, which went to her bones, and survived nearly a decade. But Karen's had gone to her bones and her liver. Karen's father's pancreatic cancer had metastasized to the liver, and he was dead in months. Of course, there were always exceptions to the odds, the unique cases, and all I could do was to cheer Karen and remind her of her mother, not her father, and pray, pray, pray to a God I wasn't sure existed that she would be spared, if not cured. I reminded Karen that if Mimi, who was old and frail, could get ten years, just think what a beautiful, young, strong specimen like herself could accomplish. Her sister had breast cancer and was fine; why not Karen?

We were at our lowest spirits after our inappropriate telephone conference with Herb when, a few days later, we got a call from a doctor in Herb's oncology group, Matt Lever, who called to give us the detailed findings of the liver biopsy. While the news wasn't good (it confirmed the three lesions the CT scan had found), Matt's attitude was the opposite of Herb's. Aside from being on the phone, it pretty much fit the SPIKE model. Karen asked him the same question, "Am I dying?" But Matt had an altogether different answer. "It's a tough road ahead," he said. "But we're going to go after this cancer. We'll get 25 percent, then another 25 percent, and then make it vanish."

Those were words that Karen and I needed to hear. We both knew from the anecdotal experience of friends and patients, as well as countless stories, that attitude can affect the course of cancer in a powerful way. Karen loved Emily Dickinson's poem that reads: "'Hope' is the thing with feathers—/ That perches in the soul—/ And sings the tune without the words—/ And never stops—at all—" Our hopes kept us going, and they kept us with Herb. The fact that a fighter like Matt was in Herb's group gave me renewed confidence. After all, this was Cedars-Sinai, the gold standard in medicine. Leaving Cedars would be like dropping out of Harvard and transferring to a state college. Besides, I rationalized, Herb's absence of personality and his deplorable bedside manner didn't diminish his stature as a doctor.

Not that my doubts about the undone scans, the ungiven Tamoxifen, and the untested markers didn't still nag me. While I kept it to myself, I was simmering to a boil with Herb. I had been so delighted with this pessimist's unusual confidence that my attitude was, "If you think she's okay, then I think she's okay." I trusted him with my wife the way I trusted him with my life. Now, in that awful thing called hindsight, I was coming to see this as a gross oversight. Still, Herb was the authority, part of a highly respected group. I was getting furious, but the idea of changing horses in the middle of this stream seemed too much, especially since the horse we were riding was supposedly Triple Crown material.

Karen was immediately set up for the procedure to install a port under her clavicle to infuse the chemotherapy drugs. Having been down this hazardous road myself, I was in a good position to cheer Karen on and allay her endless fears. I liked my port by now. It was part of my body. It had given me the elixir of life. Even though I was no longer on chemo, I left it in, just in case I had to start again. To take it out, I believed, could bring me bad luck. I wanted to avoid hubris at all costs.

Oddly enough, Karen's recent liver biopsy had revealed that her liver lesions were positive for a gene called HER2/neu (Human Epithelial Growth Factor Receptor, in medical-ese) . This HER2/neu is a protein on the cancer cell membrane that, if present, serves to make the cancer more aggressive and demands a stronger chemo treatment. On Karen's initial breast biopsy in 1999, she was negative for HER2/neu. But now she was positive, diagnosed by a special stain test known as the IHC (immunohistochemical) test, and Herb, upon learning this, prescribed a toxic addition to her IV chemo cocktail called Herceptin, which is an antibody to fight this protein. Despite the start of nausea, mouth sores, diarrhea, and hair loss, Karen was tolerating, or at least bravely surviving, her other chemo drugs.

It made no sense to me that the HER2/neu gene would test negative on the breast cancer, the source of the cancer, and then suddenly become positive on this cancer in the liver. I immediately went to my extensive medical library and began to research this conundrum. I quickly learned that it was extremely rare that the HER2/neu gene would change from the breast to the liver—the chances were one in a million. So I began to question whether the test for the gene had been done correctly. If Cedars Chairman Danny Kaye could die at Cedars after a botched blood transfusion, they could make other mistakes, too. I also learned via a casual conversation with a UCLA faculty doctor friend and fellow cancer survivor, that Herceptin, when used in conjunction with one of Karen's other chemo drugs, Adriamycin, was highly cardiotoxic; that is, it had engendered a high incidence of heart failure.

"What did her echocardiogram show?" the doctor asked me.

"What echocardiogram? She never had one," I replied. Herb had never really inquired about Karen's cardiac health, or any other health issues. "Karen's never had any heart problems."

"She doesn't have to be a candidate for open heart surgery to be at risk," the doctor said. "Combining those two drugs results in a synergistic effect. If Karen gets any untoward response, the only thing that might save her is a heart transplant."

Heart transplant! I felt as if I had just been stabbed in my heart. I thought of Karen's ravaged body, her liver and her bones ridldled with cancer, her hair falling out from chemo. And now the possibility of a heart transplant. I thought of *The Wizard of Oz*, of the Tin Man, without a heart. How could Herb be putting Karen at such hideous risk?

I called Herb in something of a panic. "Oh, we don't do echocardiograms at Cedars for that," he said casually, but not at all reassuringly. "Are hearts at UCLA (five miles away) that different?" I wanted to ask him, but I didn't want to be insulting. I was still somewhat inhibited by my recent past from asserting my outrage at the casual incompetence, if not negligence, I was seeing.

Instead of attacking Herb and the Cedars team, I decided simply and quietly to get a second opinion. I went to UCLA, which I usually avoided because it was a teaching hospital more than a practicing hospital. This impression was derived from hard personal experience. Some years before, I had gone to the UCLA emergency room one weekend with a high fever and pain; I pretty much knew what it was, acute prostatitis, but I wanted a culture and the proper antibiotics. The student doctors at UCLA, upon learning that I had lymphoma, wanted to admit me. I sensed they would have liked to turn me into an academic guinea pig, and I wasn't interested. So they hooked me up to an IV antibiotic drip in the corner of an essentially empty emergency room (it was 2 a.m.) and left me there. Eventually the drip ended, but no one came to unhook me. I called out (there was no phone) to no avail. I had been abandoned. After an hour in solitary confinement, I took the IV out myself, found some bandages to stop the bleeding, and left on my own. So much for UCLA, despite its being only minutes from my home. But now I needed that academic expertise. So I sought out Joseph Carlyle, who had written endless articles and books on breast cancer.

Finding Carlyle on the UCLA campus was no easy matter. His office, at the Jonsson Cancer Center, sits amidst an incomprehensible maze of red brick buildings with all the charm of a Russian gulag. And nobody can help with directions, because nobody seems to know where anything is. I was half an hour late, but Carlyle, a craggy English gent, was very cordial and forgiving. Unwilling to condemn his fellow cancer giant Herb Bloomfield, Carlyle did suggest a FISH test, which was a more definitive assay for the HER gene than the IHC test. FISH stood for fluorescent in situ hybridization, but I didn't care about the boring details. All I wanted was not to kill my wife in the process of trying to heal her.

Karen did the FISH test at Cedars, and the test came back negative, confirming that the original test on her breast a year ago was correct and the recent IHC stain test was wrong. I confronted Herb with this report. I told him that, given this negative result, we should stop the deadly Herceptin. I said I wasn't going to bring Karen for her Herceptin infusion the next day. "Whatever," was all he said. It was as if I was telling him I wasn't taking Karen to Disneyland. Herb didn't seem at all upset that the Cedars lab had made a major mistake that, compounded with not giving Karen an echocardiogram, might have ended her already tenuous life.

The pathologist who had read, or misread, the IHC stain test from the liver biopsy was quite upset, however. The young doctor looked at her papers and literally gasped. She was mortified with embarrassment. She said the sample piece of tissue from which she had done the IHC stain was way too small to make a definitive diagnosis of the HER2/neu gene as positive, which she had. This was "misleading," she said, which for a doctor is a major admission of having screwed up, kind of an "oops" magnified a thousand fold. The doctor graciously admitted her mistake.

Then I called the pathologist who had done the FISH test and asked him to review it once again. He took a very long moment to read Karen's chart. The silence seemed endless. Then I heard another gasp. "Wow!" the doctor exclaimed. "I can't believe this."

"Believe what?" I pressed him.

"The test was done on normal tissue," he said, with the deepest chagrin. I was beyond shocked to discover that the FISH test was as wrong as the IHC test had been; it had been done on a portion of the liver that contained normal cells, rather than on one of Karen's three cancerous growths. Jesus, I wailed to myself. Cedars-Sinai Hospital to the stars was more like a Three Stooges tragedy of errors.

Not knowing who to trust, I went into massive research mode, calling top doctors at Memorial Sloan Kettering in New York, the National Institutes of Health, the National Cancer Institute, the MD Anderson Cancer Center in Houston, Harvard, Yale, and Duke. The doctors I spoke to were all amazed and horrified by what I told them.

I had to get to the truth, and I had to be sure Karen was not further endangered by all this massive incompetence. Maybe, my mind raced, she didn't even have cancer at all. Maybe that was a misdiagnosis, too. It happens all the time, which I hadn't really believed until then.

I learned from all my queries that the FISH test had been invented right in my own backyard, by a distinguished South African doctor at the University of Southern California named Robin Levy. So I decided to go directly to the source. I called Levy up. His secretary said he was in Switzerland. I wrote him off, at least for a few weeks. Then, lo and behold, the next day Levy called me from Switzerland and couldn't have been kinder. He was on his way to Japan for an international breast cancer conference, but set up a meeting for the day he would return. Bringing Karen and all of her records, including her pathology specimens, with me, we proceeded to the eighth floor of the Norris Building of USC and found a real doctor in a real lab, full of Bunsen burners and test tubes and experiments in progress. This lovely doctor, the embodiment of the term "mensch," arranged for Karen to have another FISH test there, sampling the true cancerous liver tissue. We had to be sure.

After all the sturm und drang, a few days later I called Levy, whose first words were, "The FISH test's negative." He then proceeded to go into deeply technical jargon about the testing and the results. I respectfully listened, but to make sure I had heard the bottom line correctly, I politely asked Levy if he could repeat his very first words one more time. He quickly reiterated that the test was negative and in the same breath said, "Now you can have a nice day." I wanted to reach across the phone lines and hug the man. No preamble, no pomposity, no jargon, just health and love. The bottom line was that Karen was as negative as she had been the year before. Nothing had changed, except our frazzled psyches. Cedars' ineptitude and Herb's indifference had sent us on a debilitating wild goose chase.

If this had been a *Keystone Cops* comedy it may have been amusing, but these series of blunders were deadly. I went to the library and to my new home computer. I quickly learned that Google is a passkey to knowledge and not just a funny expression.

I found out that there are two separate issues in breast cancer treatment. The first is local: the surgery to take out the tumor. The second is systemic: the chemotherapy, which is referred to as adjuvant (or additional), to treat microscopic or metastatic disease. This therapy has toxic effects on normal cells and tissue but is more toxic to cancer cells. These cytotoxic drugs are considered poisons. They work by interfering with different aspects of the cancer cell's ability to reproduce and are used in combinations for more maximum effect. These drugs also injure normal rapidly dividing tissues like hair follicles, mouth and gutlining cells, as well as bone marrow, which produces white and red blood cells. Thus side effects can and do usually occur, including hair thinning or total loss, nausea, vomiting, mouth sores, and changes in appetite and bowel habits. Some of the drugs cause organ-specific complications including heart damage, aching of muscles and joints, neurotoxicity with tingling of fingers and toes, as well as fatigue and depression.

With this brief knowledge in mind, we re-entered the world of chemotherapy. Karen started on what would be multiple cycles of treatment sessions in the infusion room. These sessions lasted about four hours. Karen would sit in a large, grayish-pink vinyl chair that tilted back so you could go to sleep. There was no television or VCR to divert attention from the overhanging intravenous drip of the life-giving but poisonous substances. The other patients hooked up to the IVs dozed or read or simply stared into space.

The infusions were given by specially trained nurses. There was nothing particularly painful about the treatment itself. The chemicals infused through Karen's portacath were yellow or red. The red color of the adriamycin reminded Karen of a brave red warrior, a super hero with bulging muscles and a powerful piercing stare. The yellow of the taxotere represented a beautiful fairy in a glimmering gown, smiling and reassuring us that the cancer would not come back.

Karen's will to live was palpable. She refused to entertain the possibility that she would not survive. "The thing that I hate most about the chemo is losing my hair," she said. All her hair, including scalp, face, eyebrows, eyelashes, and body hair, including from private parts, was slowly but steadily lost. She made a decision that she was not a "wig type." At first she tied a scarf around her head. She said she felt like a little girl when she stood in the shower looking down at her hairless crotch. She stopped looking down. We often wrote notes to each other, and hers she would sign "Baldy." After tiring of seeing the hair fall out, she went to her fabulous Beverly Hills hairdresser, Shahrzad, and underwent hair cutting magic. She became a gorgeous Mia Farrow look-alike. Her radically shortened hair made the transition to Miss Baldy a lot easier.

In the chemo lounge, or fusion room, we heard some stories. A lady across from us said that the more wretched she felt after treatment, the more she knew the chemo was working. Some of her best hours of hope and optimism were spent with her head in the toilet. Sitting in that room, a place I had known just three years before, I realized how cancer pulls you out of the false sense of security that you are guaranteed to grow old. According to all that was written about NHL, my period of complete remission was coming to an end. I told myself I had to remain viable to be with Karen in this journey—this cancer journey.

As if I didn't have enough problems, I was blindsided by a letter from the California Medical Board that my license to practice medicine was being suspended in light of my conviction. I was summoned to medical board offices in Riverside, in the Inland Empire, on the way to Palm Springs. Karen, sick as she was, insisted on going with me. I wanted to spare her this humiliation, but she wouldn't hear it. Tim Pool went with us. We had never even discussed the possibility of suspension; we were too busy thinking about San Quentin. The suspension was another kick in the teeth.

There is nothing even vaguely imperial about Riverside, which used to be a capital of an empire of citrus groves, now mostly depleted, and is now a capital of smog and auto repairs. Karen waited in the barren anteroom as Tim and I proceeded into the lion's den of State Assistant Attorney General Andy Berger. Berger was a fat, jovial Falstaff of a guy, except his news was anything but jolly. The board, according to California law, had no choice but to suspend me. At the moment, I didn't really care. Karen's cancer had me totally obsessed anyhow, and I had yet to begin to rebuild my practice. This was fine. I would be Karen's doctor, and only hers. But then the humiliation hit me, and the flood of emotions from my cancer and Karen's, and I somehow lost it. I suddenly began to weep uncontrollably. How ignominious could it get for the golden boy from the Bronx? Tim took me out of the room and, with Karen's help, tried to calm me down with a pep talk of the kind a trainer would give a boxer on the ropes. I had to control myself,

Tim ordered me. Real men didn't cry. Don't show weakness, or they'll punish you more, just as dogs bite people who show fear.

I finally pulled it together, but it wasn't as necessary as Tim had thought. Karen went back into Berger's office with me, and he was instantly smitten with her, not to mention being deeply moved by her cancer and my commitment to caring for her. Andy Berger was no mean dog, but rather the rare nice government lawyer. "You're way too nice to be in the justice system," Karen told him, kind of flirtatiously but in all sincerity, given what she had seen me going through. Andy loved it, loved her, and started to like me. Andy began talking about his own problems with sleep apnea, how his state insurance company wouldn't allow him to see an ENT specialist. Hey, Karen, said, you've got that specialist right in front of you.

After composing myself, I threw out some suggestions Andy hadn't heard before, and his ears pricked up. He was wowed by my thorough approach, my diagnostic and treatment ideas, off the cuff as they were. He saw that I cared, and apparently his other doctors had not. Had the simple virtue of caring become that rare? It was a sad commentary on the profession that had just censured me.

Within an hour Andy, Karen, and I had totally bonded, and within a half hour more, Andy was conceding I had gotten the rawest of deals. We talked about the current scandal in the U.S. Attorney's Office, the office that had prosecuted me. The head of that office, Alejandro Mayorkas, it had been discovered, had lobbied the recently departed President Clinton, who had appointed him, to grant an end-of-term pardon to a major drug kingpin named Carlos Vignali. Clinton had come under heavy fire for these pardons, beginning with fugitive financier Marc Rich, who had once owned Twentieth Century Fox before evading millions in taxes over very shady oil deals with Iran and Iraq. But as bewildering as the Rich pardon was, the Vignali one was far more incomprehensible. Vignali was the key figure in a massive crack cocaine ring, the profits of which were so great that he would routinely gamble hundreds of thousands of it away on lost weekends in Las Vegas. High living for a guy whose tax return declared he only earned $30,000 slaving away at his father's auto body repair shop.

Vignali and his ring had been convicted. Vignali himself was serving a fifteen year sentence. But his father, Horacio, whose auto business was a huge one, began donating money, big money, to leading California politicians. Why Mayorkas, a Democrat and a self-professed law-and-order guy who had decreed the witch hunt on me, would have sullied himself by lobbying his boss, President Clinton, for Vignali was way beyond me and beyond lawman Andy as well. Eventually Mayorkas would resign, certainly in part over this scandal. He, too, conceded, "I made a mistake. I felt some compassion for the father (the multimillionaire influence peddler who had been a federal suspect in the narcotics trade for over twenty years) and regrettably, that compassion may have been misplaced." Where was that compassion when a basically innocent doctor with terminal cancer came before his office? I wondered. The hypocrisy of Mayorkas was an outrage to everyone, especially me, a victim of it, and to Karen, whose acute sense of fairness might be said to be Solomonic.

Andy exhorted me to put the injustices of the past behind me, and to follow his steps to do a quick penance to the med board through a series of required exams and workshops to prove my character wasn't fatally flawed. He felt I could get my license reinstated quickly, and he promised to help me in whatever way he could. He was so impressed by my resume and the way I talked about his condition with him that he blurted out, "You should be practicing medicine, Dr. Reiter. That's where you belong." That vote of confidence helped me regain my full license a few months later and have maintained it since. But right then I wasn't thinking of myself and my own professional future. I was only thinking about trying to save the woman I loved, who had just saved the day, and perhaps my medical future, for me. License or no license, I was still a doctor and I would devote every skill I had to Karen.

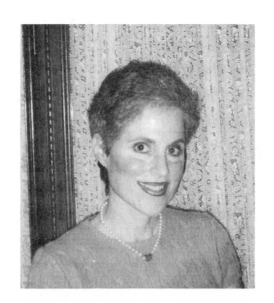

Karen after chemo

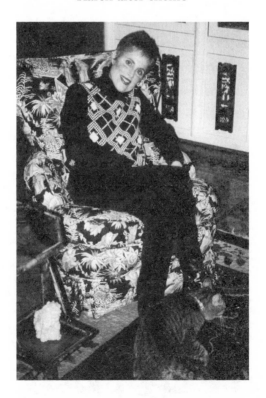

Chapter Ten

THE DOCTOR, IN SPITE OF HIMSELF

While Karen began her chemotherapy, I began my community service, which was part of my court-ordered penance. Both of us suffered, in very different ways. Karen had dreadful experiences with fever, nausea, diarrhea, total loss of hair, loss of taste, and a deep depression. Here was a beautiful woman, ravaged, defeminized, brought down low. She received no counseling as to what to expect during chemo. She was never even advised to see a dentist, in spite of the fact that it is highly recommended to visit a dentist at least three weeks before chemotherapy. Chemotherapy creates inflammation of the mouth, and a small problem such as a tooth cavity before chemo can become a big one during treatment. We were never prepared to deal with the many known side effects of these poisons. Luckily Karen's sixth sense, and her pride in her dazzling smile, led her to consult a dentist. If she had followed Herb's non-advice, she could have had big mouth trouble.

After several months, Karen's tumor marker numbers began to decline, albeit less precipitously than the NASDAQ that year. Like most investors, I would lose a great deal of paper profits as the tech

265

bubble burst, but I didn't care. What mattered to me was my wife. Cancer does force you to get your priorities straight.

What also mattered to me was my profession, and to be excluded from it caused me a profound melancholy and unremitting sadness, compounded by the specter of losing Karen. If I didn't have my livelihood or my true love, what would there be to continue living for? Right now I did have Karen, and my mission was to save her, to hell with the odds. I deeply resented having to spend any time away from her, particularly in connection with my legal punishment, which I increasingly came to view as justice of the kangaroo court variety. Still, I had more than one hundred hours of community service to complete, pretty much at my own discretion, so I decided to devote them to fighting the lymphoma that I had thus far battled successfully.

Back during the darkest days of my own illness, in 1998, I had joined, somewhat tentatively at first, a support group at UCLA for people with blood diseases such as lymphoma, leukemia, and multiple myeloma. I had done it without fanfare, because Karen didn't believe in such groups, even in her own darkest hours. She believed a true lady or gentleman should keep his or her disease to him or herself. Maybe she got this attitude from her beloved English literature, which generally extolled the virtues of the stiff upper lip. Her reluctance to join such groups notwithstanding, her own devotion to Weight Watchers was cultish in its intensity. But that was different, she said; it was purely practical and goal-oriented. Maybe Karen had her own spiritual core and didn't need the input of others. I myself was a little abashed that I eventually found a lot of comfort in the kindness of strangers.

While Karen was on chemo, I went with her to a Chinese manicurist. The woman, a wise old philosopher type, urged Karen to attend a support group, like the Wellness Community for Breast Cancer. "I don't want to hear their stories," Karen said.

"At least there are people there who can tell their stories," the manicurist said, and I blurted out, "Confucius has nothing over you, Mei Ling." I saw in her the embodiment of Chinese spirituality, and I recalled the wonderful proverb, "To know the road ahead, ask those coming back." People who have been through cancer generally have a special bond with one another. I suggested to Karen that she heed the lesson I'd learned, that sharing what you've been through with others and hearing how they coped with problems like your own can be a great source of strength. But Karen was strong on her own, and even Lady Confucius couldn't sway her. "I've got Alvin," Karen parried, jokingly and proudly.

I myself needed all the help I could get. I remember my first group meeting when I introduced myself and said what I did and what kind of cancer I had. The reaction of the group surprised me. They didn't seem to think that as a doctor I needed to be there because I already knew everything, but also, they were rather shocked that a doctor actually got sick. They seemed to think I had access to a higher level of care, like insider trading, that would allow me to beat all scourges and simply fade away at the ripest of old ages. I explained that I was both a doctor and a patient, and was just like them. But they never quite believed it. I had a great deal of stature among them, and it was with the deepest shame after my conviction that I had to approach Kathleen York, the saintly oncologic social worker who ran the group, and tell her that I was now a felon who needed her help.

As I nearly choked on my own words, Kathleen herself broke down in tears. "What a waste, what a waste," she wailed, bemoaning the injustice of any system that could do this to someone she knew was such a good and giving group member. "This shouldn't have happened to you. You're such a fine person," she told me after I bore my secret to her.

"How do you know I'm such a fine person?" I asked, not wanting to believe my own good reviews.

"I know you. I know you," was all she could say. I was flattered that she really understood the man behind the medical degree.

Her benedictions aside, Kathleen consulted with her UCLA colleagues and got them to authorize my community service there, performing a wide range of functions from arranging private nursing care for cancer patients at home, to organizing reams of literature from every medical school on the newest treatments. For years as I sat in the group I had watched in bemusement as patients brought up all these new clinical trials at Harvard, Johns Hopkins, Beijing, wherever, hoping against any realistic hope that some researcher somewhere would discover a magic bullet for their illness.

Why, I used to think to myself, didn't they just trust their doctors, who were up on everything and spare themselves this ordeal of false encouragement. Little did I know that Karen's illness would soon drive me to far greater extremes. I had been a great believer in, and respecter of, doctors. I deferred to authority. That's how I was trained. And that's why I deferred to Dexter, and look what that had gotten me. In any event, I finished my hundred hours of community service in a month and a half. I was relearning that giving, in this case giving my time to counsel fellow NHL cancer travelers, was so much more rewarding than receiving that I continued to work with Kathleen as a volunteer.

Karen's chemo ended in January 2001. Most of the year was devoted to her recovery, her return to the land of the living. Karen's tumor marker had changed dramatically from 15 (a normal score) in October 1999 to 115 almost a year later. This tumor marker blood test, the CA 15-3, is a significant barometer of cancer. Each month we waited with high anxiety for the results of her blood tests, and each time we breathed sighs of relief when the tumor marker numbers were lower.

It indicated whether she would live or die and for how long she would survive. The blood was drawn the morning of her chemotherapy and the results were back the next morning, although most patients only got them a week later on a subsequent office visit. Waiting is one of the worst parts of the cancer experience. A doctor may have a hundred things to do each day, but for the patient waiting at home for the test results, each minute can be an eternity, as this is the most important thing in his or her life. Luckily, as a doctor I was granted some privileges, including being able to call the lab the next day. With a deep breath and a deeper sense of dread I would ask, "Do you have the results of Karen Reiter's CA 15-3 tumor marker? Yes…I'll hold." An eternity went by until that disembodied voice came back and announced the result. "It's sixty-two, Dr. Reiter." Another drop in the numbers, not yet in the normal range but going in the right direction. (Thirty or under was the promised land.) While these tests were only part of the picture, I was grateful for the smallest mercies.

But that spring something wonderful happened. "The number is 19.6, Dr. Reiter." I made the disembodied voice repeat the number. "It's 19.6, Dr. Reiter." It had been forty-five the month before. Now we were well within the under-thirty zone, from 115 to 93 to 86 to 75 to 62, 45, and now 19.6. Valhalla! Karen could detect my enthusiasm, make that joy, as I bounded up the stairs. "Forget the NASDAQ, Dow Jones, S&P, day of the week, your birthday. This is your lucky number!"

I had written it on a white piece of cardboard and held it high, just like an Olympic scorecard. "Cherish it!' I shouted, and we hugged and cried and laughed. That number, on that piece of cardboard, was our own cross against the vampire of cancer. Cancer, begone! A multitude of other tests added to our hope, showing Karen's liver lesions had shrunk, and that there were no new growths. Furthermore, the chemo had worked so well that her bone lesions had disappeared. More sighs of relief, if only until the next test.

But in September, right after the horrible events of 9/11, our briefly happy little world began to be terrorized as well. Karen's tumor marker level began to rise again, to twenty-six, the edge of normal. "That's a bad sign," Karen said, invoking her sixth sense. "It's just a number," I countered, invoking my inner New Yorker. I should have known better than to gainsay Karen's "signs" because sure enough, by October, the tumor marker was thirty-six, the edge of abnormal. The scans remained good, but the direction of the numbers was bad.

That winter, Kathleen asked me to address the third-year class at UCLA Medical School on the subject of a doctor as cancer survivor as well as a cancer caregiver, my personal story. Karen came with me as Exhibit A. For two-and-a-half hours we sat on stage and were interviewed by a psychologist and a psychiatrist. They asked all the right questions of me and Karen, questions from the heart, asked with grace, courtesy, and curiosity, both factual and spiritual queries that brought us in touch with each other. We occupied two chairs on the podium but spoke as one.

We related how we felt that cancer was an emotional albatross, always there even when it was temporarily gone. Looking out from the podium, I could see Cancer walking in and taking a front-row seat in this absurd theatre of our lives that happened to be a UCLA auditorium. I shared with all these bright and hopeful young students how cancer had jolted me out of my false sense of security that I was guaranteed to grow old. I spoke of my new sense of optimism of not dying of cancer but living with cancer. It was an optimism of reduced expectations, but this was reality, and these were big boys and girls who needed to hear the truth of my life lesson.

Toward the end of this powerful, draining session, I looked at my lovely Karen, obviously worn down by her relentless battle with this malignancy, and said that I had become a doctor in 1970 and that if I never practiced again, I was still happy that I had become a doctor to be able to help my wife. The whole class got out their handkerchiefs.

There wasn't a dry eye in the auditorium.

I was working full time trying to figure out a way to beat Karen's cancer. Now that it was confined to the liver, and was nowhere else to be found in her body, I asked myself, what more can we do to get rid of it, or at least control it? I would spend every day either in the UCLA medical library or going to lectures and oncology meetings in the LA area. Sometimes I traveled around the state and country, learning the state of the cancer art. The treatments of choice of the top oncologists in the field, from Harvard, Yale, Duke, and Stanford, all of whom I tracked down and either buttonholed at meetings or called on the phone, were two procedures: the first was Radiofrequency Ablation, or RFA, in which the liver tumors were burned away; and the second was "resection," in which the cancerous parts of the liver were cut away and the remaining liver sewn back together. The procedures were often combined.

Not a single doctor I pursued turned me down. They were all ears, all sympathy, and they all wanted to see me get results that would benefit all of us. Medicine was a common good, and I was inspired by the way these great doctors stepped up to my challenge. Some doctors were harder to reach than others. The toughest was Peter Greco, the chief of surgical oncology at UCLA, a very grand and distant man. One day at UCLA I saw him across a huge lobby at a bank of elevators, and I rushed to stop him before the doors slammed shut. He was highly annoyed at me, but as soon as I said the magic words, "My wife has metastatic breast cancer spread to the liver," he got out of the elevator and lent me his ears. To my pleasant surprise, he escorted me to his office, closed the door, and asked me to sit down. He urged me to tell him my story, all of it, and he made me feel that I had his undivided attention (rare for a doctor, whose attention is always divided) and that Karen was the only sick person he was thinking about.

I mentioned to Greco a Cedars liver surgeon named Michael Greaves whom Herb had recommended. As it turned out, Greaves had been a student of Greco's while he was training at UCLA. Greco gave him the thumbs-up, assuring me that Greaves was well-trained and very capable of doing liver cancer surgery, although we did not discuss the RFA part of the procedure I had been contemplating for Karen. If the renowned Peter Greco said Greaves was a good man, he was good enough for me.

In February 2002, Karen and I had our first consultation with Michael Greaves (pronounced "graves"), widely lauded as the cutting-edge liver surgeon at Cedars. Greaves was in his early forties, Australian, and extremely skeletal. There was nothing of the robust, shrimp-on-the-barbie Aussie footballer. He was more like Klaus Barbie, a very scary undertaker sort of guy. But, hey, geniuses weren't supposed to look like Crocodile Dundee. He was at Cedars, which was like a Good

Housekeeping Seal of Approval. Even in Los Angeles, there weren't a plethora of great liver surgeons, so our options were limited.

We talked to Greaves about a surgical procedure that involved opening the abdomen and resecting, or cutting away, all three of Karen's liver tumors. This had been the advice given to us at a consultation a few weeks before with a liver surgeon at City of Hope Hospital, a major Southern California cancer center. Then we discussed radiofrequency ablation, or RFA. This procedure used a high frequency current to burn the tumor cells to death. The gold standard for treatment of malignant liver tumors remained resection, but I had read that RFA could be used in combination with surgical resection for tumors that would otherwise be deemed unresectable. In RFA a thin wire, or electrode, is placed into the liver. The zone of tissue death is limited, and the procedure needs to be repeated numerous times during the same surgery not only to encompass the actual cancerous lesion but also to obtain a margin of safety to ensure that all of the tumor is destroyed as well. Such margins are a general principle of cancer treatment, whether it be RFA, surgery, or radiation.

We then talked to Greaves about a surgical procedure that involved both excision and RFA, in which Karen's three liver tumors would basically be both cut and burned away. It was a drastic measure, but cancer is a drastic disease, and Karen was used to drastic measures at this point. The key thing was that the measures succeed, and Greaves indicated that Karen was a prime candidate for this procedure. Karen, as seen by her double mastectomy, was as decisive as General Patton when it came to her health. She wasn't going to just sit back and watch that tumor marker rise until it was too late. She wanted to live, and would do whatever it took. Accordingly, we set a surgery date for early April 2002.

As I sat there with yet one more cancer doctor, I recalled a quotation that helped me summon up the faith that I desperately needed now: "When you come to the edge of all that you know, you must believe in one of two things: there will be earth upon which to stand, or you will be given wings to fly." (Author unknown, but attribution didn't matter to me.)

I thought of Paul Donald, the oddsmaker, the great surgeon I had trained under at UC Davis, and it turned out that Greaves knew him. At the risk of seeming preachy and pedantic, I couldn't stop myself from telling Greaves the most important lesson I had learned from Donald, which was that, no matter how hopeless a case might look, a doctor should do all he can, despite the odds, because the patient's life is in the doctor's hands. I didn't sense that Greaves resented my telling this story. I didn't mean to lecture him or hector him on how to live his life as a doctor; in fact, I assumed he was as dedicated as I was. Yet with the errors at Cedars, with Herb's gloomy, write-her-off negativity, I needed to give voice to my own compulsiveness that Karen get the best, most passionate care there was.

A few weeks before Karen's April surgery, at Kathleen's request, I served as a volunteer at the American Cancer Society's "Daffodil Days," held at the UCLA Cancer Clinic. The idea was that daffodils were a symbol of spring and of hope, and my task was to hand out these flowers to all the visitors and patients to the clinic to raise their awareness of cancer research. We wanted everyone's involvement in the cause to make the world free from cancer. This medical rite of spring was inspired by the Wordsworth poem, "I Wandered Lonely as a Cloud." Karen, who loved Wordsworth and his cherished Lake District, knew the poem by heart:

I wandered lonely as a cloud
That floats on high o'er vales and hills,
When all at once I saw a crowd,
A host, of golden daffodils;
Beside the lake, beneath the trees,
Fluttering and dancing in the breeze…
…The waves beside them danced; but they
Out-did the sparkling waves in glee:
A poet could not but be gay,
In such a jocund company:
I gazed—and gazed—but little thought
What wealth the show to me had brought…

At first I somehow resented the idea of a once-proud surgeon becoming a flower boy. I felt I should have been inside the UCLA Hospital treating the patients, not outside handing out daffodils. What a waste, as Kathleen had said. But Karen, notwithstanding her disinclination toward group activities, offered to come with me and give out daffodils, too. It was unspoken that we probably weren't going to be visiting Windermere and Grassmere or any of those idyllic English towns in the foreseeable future. The UCLA campus, bursting with spring flowers, was as close to the Lake District as we were going to get. Karen, always positive, forced me to make the most of it.

As I handed out flowers, I felt a little like Albert Brooks in his comedy *Lost in America*, when he played a fallen business hotshot reduced to serving as a school crossing guard. But I got over it, especially when I saw the joy each patient received from getting those daffodils. Soon I got into it, giving a mini-sermon to each person on the beauty of spring, how hope "springs" eternal, how I was a doctor who was surviving cancer. After my initial rush of anger about the injustice of my own precipitous fall from grace, sharing my story and my emotions made me feel lucky to be there.

As I was unwrapping daffodils and putting them in vases, a distraught woman with a heavy foreign accent came up to me for a flower. She told me that she was there with her husband, who had NHL, my cancer. Surrendering my own privacy, I became myself, the doctor-patient, not the flower volunteer, and briefly shared my story. It perked her up. She then showed me her husband, who was slumped over on a distant bench and looked like death warmed over. She said her husband was from Spain and barely spoke English, and how sad it was that he couldn't hear my story from me.

I got the bright idea to enlist Karen's help. I knew how she felt about self-help conclaves and I knew she was facing major cancer surgery, but I also knew she loved people and was a natural partner to anyone in distress, so I asked her if she could translate for me, and, of course, she rose to the occasion, giving him a shot of hope by telling the man how I had survived eight years with this disease. Karen was so kind and compassionate, in her elegant Castilian accent, that she reminded me of Dame Cicely Saunders, the all-giving, deeply Christian British nurse, and later doctor, who founded the Hospice movement in England in the 1960s. It was that movement that gave rise to the concept of palliative as opposed to curative, care, and profoundly enhanced the dignity of the end of life when modern medicine, in its quest for "victories" and "cures," had given up.

"Palliative" had been derived from the Greek, meaning "to cloak over," or conceal. The word had developed over the years to refer to a means of alleviating symptoms without eliminating the disease itself, to relieve, reduce, or soothe these symptoms to achieve the best quality of life, as long as that life could go on. Hospice was derived from the Latin "hospis," or host, as in caring for guests. That word evolved from receiving weary travelers, or pilgrims, to a place of welcome and care for those in acute need, i.e., the sick and dying. Because modern medicine has focused on curative treatments and not holistic care—care for the soul, nurture of the mind and spirit—honor and care for the dying has inevitably been displaced. Dame Cicely noted this neglect. This was her manifesto: "You matter until the last moment of your life. We will do all we can not only to help you die peacefully but also to live until you die." So here was Dame Cicely, Mother Teresa, and Florence Nightingale, all in one, Saint Karen. She would have been amazing in the group meetings, a beacon to all, if only she had come. The Spanish man's countenance changed from night to day after Karen finished talking with him; it was as if she had healed him.

Later on, I gave my sermon-on-the-mount, along with a handful of daffodils, to a distinguished older woman who, to my eye, didn't look sick or grieving, as everyone else at the clinic did. I was right. "Do you know who I am?" the dowager asked. I said that I didn't. "Young man," she said, in a Katherine Hepburn voice, "I am the president of the Los Angeles chapter of the American Cancer Society, and I must say I've been watching you, and what you are doing is remarkable. You are marvelous!" I was so inspired by her praise that I envisioned myself taking my message on the road all over the country to all those, like myself, who were not really cured but not really dying either, the limbo rock of cancer. More important, I was inspired that I had a certain power to heal still within me. This flower boy was still a doctor, through and through.

There were some very anxious moments leading up to Karen's operation. We went to Herb not for his blessing but for a medical evaluation, standard prior to surgery. After his usual laconic greeting and a cursory review of Karen's past and present medical history, he performed a perfunctory physical examination. Fortunately, this was not crucial, as Karen had had every nook and cranny of her body examined and reexamined over the past year. Herb cleared her for the impending surgery. But, as a parting shot, instead of a simple "good-bye and good luck," he did something neither of us would ever forget, or forgive. Directly to Karen's face, he said, "You know, Karen, you will not be cured by this surgery." Then, as if to plunge the knife in even more deeply, he added, "And you'll have a big scar, a really big scar," and swept his hand, as if he were making the incision, across her entire abdomen. Karen stared at him in disbelief. I wanted to hurl him out the window, at the very least.

Dr. Francis Peabody, one of America's greatest physicians and educators, wrote in 1927, "The secret of the care of the patient is in caring for the patient." If Herb did not care about his patients, he should not have been in medicine, no matter how brilliant he may have been. How cruel, how brutal. This wasn't doctor behavior, unless the doctor was Mengele. As my mother, who had no medical degree but abundant common sense, always said, "If you don't have anything nice to say, don't say anything at all."

Greaves, the liver surgeon, had scheduled no pre-op appointment, so Karen herself called for one. Greaves' secretary told her it wasn't indicated and that Greaves didn't "do" them, he was terribly busy doing "real" surgery, and he couldn't talk to her today because he was rushing out to attend the funeral of a very important patient. To Karen, a reader of omens, that was a very ominous one indeed. Maybe Greaves was not the surgeon we should choose.

We both knew that it is standard procedure to see the surgeon before the surgery. This was just not theory to us; it's the way we practiced for over twenty years. In a quiet, undisturbed setting, the surgeon, in a time-honored position, discusses with the patient her medical diagnosis, the aims of the proposed surgery, what to expect in the initial and then later post-op period, and last and perhaps most important of all, surgical complications.

This is called an informed consent. It is a statement of fidelity between the surgeon and the patient upon whom the surgery is to be performed. It represents a canon of loyalty. Karen knew from her experience running our office that when a fully informed person consents to a procedure or treatment, doctor and patient are in agreement about the goal and the means toward its achievement. Not to proceed with all the parts goes directly against the canons of medical ethics.

But Karen was decisive about this surgery and wanted to stay the course. My research and multiple consultations with doctors and medical cancer institutions across the county had led me to believe that this proposed liver surgery including RFA was the best option out of a very limited choice of options. Karen and I both felt that the alternative of doing nothing, as Herb had advocated, was a non-option; that would be to give up without a fight. The old saying still held, where there is life, there is hope, at least for a significant remission.

Greaves was a board-certified liver surgeon, trained at UCLA, and he was a member of the liver transplant team at Cedars. After our many pleading phone calls, he finally agreed to see us. It was just three days before the surgery in the early evening. Basically, he said, Karen had nothing to worry about. Because Karen was the one with the sixth sense, if she had wanted to pull the plug on Greaves, I would have seconded her decision. But she wanted to go ahead with it.

Right before Karen's surgery, I had a thought, about the possible use or value of the liver specimen that would be removed in surgery. I knew a portion would be put in formaldehyde for diagnoses and to determine if clear margins of normal tissue were obtained surrounding the cancer. I had a feeling that part of the specimen needed to be saved and not embalmed, as it would be in formaldehyde. Deep in my heart, I felt perhaps, with preservation, further tests could be run, if not now, then in the future, to stave off this cancer monster. I was aware that stem cells could be kept alive for future use in transplant procedures. But what about cancer cells? Certainly not to transplant to another human being. While I didn't know exactly why a specimen should be saved, it was a thought I couldn't dismiss.

It finally dawned on me that specimens can be kept alive in a solution of liquid nitrogen, the same solution that dermatologists use to freeze and remove superficial skin lesions. Formaldehyde kills tissue; liquid nitrogen keeps it alive. Liquid nitrogen is stored in a small container like a coffee thermos. I called the pathology lab at Cedars to see about putting some of Karen's prospective liver specimens in this solution. The pathologist I spoke with refused to do it. This guy was an embalmer, not a life preserver. He talked on and on about the many layers of approval and committees that would have to be navigated, and how they would need the blessings of every major medical and cancer institution in the country as well as the approval of the president of the United States. I protested to no avail. Formaldehyde is like embalming fluid, not a preservative, I protested. God, I despaired, the

Cedars pathology department, which had put me through hell before, was beyond pathological.

I called Dr. Joseph Carlyle and Dr. Paul Herman at their UCLA offices and left long messages with their secretaries as well as on their voice mails. I also contacted other departments of oncology. I really didn't have a clear idea what I wanted done with the samples if I got approved, but I just felt it was necessary. Paul Herman returned my call before the surgery. "Of course we can put it in liquid nitrogen," he said. "We do it all the time. All we need is running water, electricity, and a three-inch shelf space for the thermos. Couldn't be simpler." I thanked him very much and he wished the best for Karen. Dr. Herman was known nationwide and internationally as a leading authority on NHL. He was also known as one of the kindest, gentlest, most caring physicians around. I couldn't help but have the morbid thought that if my own NHL came back, he was the guy I would call.

The same day, before Karen went in for surgery, amidst all the trauma of getting ready to go to the hospital, I got a call from one Dr. Sylvan Minsky, a breast cancer pathologist at UCLA who had heard about Karen's upcoming liver cancer surgery from my UCLA friend Joseph Carlyle. It was 3 p.m. Minsky wanted to know how he could help me, so I told him the whole story up to then, in staccato form. As if in answer to my vague sense of posterity, he asked me if I could get him one of those pieces of Karen's liver I had been trying so hard to preserve. His idea was to try to create a xenograft, which means injecting and growing Karen's cancer cells in mice. Sure, I said. Anything for science. I had no idea why exactly Minsky wanted to do this, but before he could explain it to me, our phone connection got filled with static. He said he would call me right back. He didn't.

At that point, I called the chairman of the Cedars pathology department. I wanted to tell him that I felt he had three criminals masquerading as pathologists, but I was so surprised he actually got on the phone that I was polite. I was even more surprised that he agreed with me about liquid nitrogen and readily gave his assent to taking the sample to Minsky at UCLA. Given my experience with Cedars pathology, I assumed that everything would go wrong, that the samples would be preserved incorrectly, that they would rot on a lab table, that they wouldn't be delivered in time, but I accepted the chairman's effusive assurances that all would proceed by the letter.

At around 9:00 p.m., Minsky called back, to my surprise. I filled him in on the complete course of Karen's illness, a narrative I had to go through with every new specialist I consulted. Minsky outlined to me how he would take the liver specimen, inject it into a mouse, and develop a xenograft, a growth from human to rodent. Then he added the kicker: I must provide him with consent to do this procedure.

I told him we were at home, it was late, but I could send the consent in the morning along with the liver specimen. I would give you a pint of my blood if you want, I thought, but why do you need a consent for this? There was a momentary pause on the line and then he said, "I may develop a cancer vaccine with this and win a Nobel Prize, and you'll be upset that you didn't give me consent!"

I thought for a moment: who is this strange man calling in what seemed to be the middle of the night, just hours before this literally life-and-death surgery? And he's going to win a Nobel Prize? The strange cancer journey had just gotten even stranger. We talked for a little while longer and he explained all the difficulties with the bureaucracy at UCLA and elsewhere and quickly told me of his work, for which he had won recognition, especially with inflammatory breast cancer. Breast cancer was his passion, and he conveyed determination to beat this fearsome disease.

I assured him the consent form would go to UCLA along with the liquid nitrogen-preserved tissue samples right after surgery. I felt I had entered an old *Twilight Zone* episode with this phantom scientist.

Karen was upstairs in the bedroom worrying about where I was and worrying about the impending surgery. I put two thumbs up. "Dr. Minsky and your liver are going to win a Nobel Prize, and you do not win it for losing propositions!" I could see her face light up. It gave her the kind of hope a patient needs on the eve of a major operation.

Karen's cancer diagnosis had forced her to the edge of life where the important things come into focus: the love of her friends and family, a sense of wonder at the world, and an ability to cherish and feel time. Karen did not have wild hopes for a miracle cure; she would not allow herself such myth-making. She hoped to continue in her state of health and stabilize. Dr. Minsky's project was as long a shot as long shots go, and that Nobel might have been years away, but it would sustain her through all her post-op miseries to come.

As I closed my eyes, I thought of the African proverb, "However long the night, the dawn will break."

The dawn did, of course, break, and at 5:00 a.m. we were off to the hospital. I accompanied Karen to pre-op holding, where she was interviewed by the anesthesiologist. I was impressed by his confidence but more so by his humanity, which calmed me. Karen and I held each other and I felt that she would be okay with the surgery and perhaps this would be a breakthrough.

At 8:30 a.m., about an hour into the surgery, the anesthesiologist called me in the waiting area to report that the liver specimen was being sent to the pathology lab and the operation was going well. I told him nervously "Please, please, it has to be sent immediately to the lab and then by fast delivery to UCLA, it's going to be injected…"

"Dr. Reiter," he interrupted, " I know, we all know…it will be taken care of."

As soon as he said, "we all know" I felt such encouragement that I had a whole team, a whole hospital, a whole university medical school, the whole world behind Karen. In my sleepless state, I thought of the disco song, "I Will Survive." Yes, Gloria Gaynor and Karen. She will survive, I vowed to myself.

Greaves came out of the OR with a smile. "NED!" he boasted, which was doctor-speak for No Evidence of Disease after the procedure. He told me how he had resected a small portion of the liver's left lateral lobe, where two of Karen's three lesions were, removing them. Then he went at the remaining lesion in the right lobe, cutting into it. But he had stopped, fearing that he might have to cut away too much of Karen's liver, thus jeopardizing her life. Then he performed RFA on that lesion, and he "got it," he said. Greaves assured me that the rest of the liver and abdomen were cancer-free and quite healthy. My reaction was concern rather than celebration. I worried that cutting into a cancer, without entirely removing it, could cause the cancer to spread. But he assured me that the RFA solved that problem and zapped that large lesion, too large to cut out, into oblivion. "NED," he repeated, and went home.

Karen remained at Cedars for the next seven days, in such hideous pain for two of the days that she required an IV Dilaudid and morphine drip. Her continued grace under the pressure of this pain never ceased to amaze me. She'd insist on getting up, brushing her teeth, washing her face, combing her hair, looking her best, always being cheerful. She was not only a domestic goddess; she was a hospital goddess. What she wasn't cheerful about was when she heard how Greaves had begun to cut into the lesion and then stopped and switched to RFA. "You don't cut into a cancer and stop," Karen said. She had read all about cancer. This admonition went back to the ancient Greeks. In 200 A.D. the great doctor Galen appreciated the value of wide removal and recommended excision through the healthy surrounding tissue. He said, "Make accurate incisions surrounding the whole tumor so as not to leave a single root."

"He spread the cancer," Karen said in disbelief. "He spread the cancer."

"No way," I declared. "He burnt the hell out of it. It's gone," I insisted. "Don't worry. It's gone."

Greaves himself stopped by only twice. The rest of the time his students and fellows came for him. Eventually Karen pulled through and was discharged. She went home, resumed her light exercises and her admirably healthy anti-oxidant, low-fat diet. Her wounds healed steadily. We went to Greaves's office two weeks later for a post-op follow-up, and he seemed eager to show us the door. Karen was still anxious about his having cut into a cancer without removing it, and her questions seemed to annoy him. We asked for a post-op scan, which he said couldn't be done before two months after the surgery.

In our endless research before meeting Greaves, Karen and I had obtained several pages of UCLA protocol prepared expressly for RFA of the liver. I recalled reading that a CT of the liver is done immediately after the RFA to assess the results and to redo the procedure if residual cancer remains. What stuck in my mind was the word "immediately."

"Who's the surgeon here?" Greaves asked, insulted that we questioned his authority. Once again, I deferred to that authority. I reminded myself that he was a liver surgeon, on the transplant team at a major hospital, and so forth, the litany of credentials doctors lived by.

"Keep your cork on," he admonished us. Karen was fine. She was feeling better; she was better. Out the door.

A month later, in mid-May, we went to see Herb. Karen's tumor marker, which was fifty-nine before the surgery, had only dropped to fifty-six. I asked Herb, after this liver surgery, why the tumor marker CA 15-3 wasn't lower. Herb became agitated and annoyed. "I told you not to have that surgery, but it's too late now. It may not be in the liver; it's probably spread elsewhere," he declared, right in her face, as if admonishing a child. Poor Karen, calm, composed, brave Karen, burst into uncontrollable tears at Herb's abject cruelty. I myself was equally appalled and totally speechless. Seeing the very heart and soul of my life shattered into pieces, I wanted to attack Herb physically. I was seconds away from homicide—justifiable homicide.

Herb's attitude was that Karen was a "dead woman walking." Why bother to prolong the inevitable? Enough was enough. Herb had a Harvard Business School efficiency expert's approach to his patients. Why waste effort on Karen, who was a bad risk, when he could spend it on someone who had a better chance to live more years than Karen did? Planned obsolescence, accelerated depreciation. These were concepts for inventory, not people. Karen and I had no choice now but to fire Herb, for his sheer inhumanity. I had lost confidence in the man who had supposedly saved my life. I realized it was luck and established standard medicine, rather than skill, that saved me. I recalled all the books that I thought were overly critical of modern medicine, books with tabloid titles like *How to Survive Your Doctor's Care, Wall of Silence: The Untold Story of the Medical Mistakes that Kill and Injure Millions of*

Americans, and *I'm Alive and the Doctor's Dead*, books I would now read with more respect. This was the bitter end of what I had hoped would be a splendid, triumphant relationship.

For all her tears, for all her pain, Karen never lost her grace. Here is the letter she wrote to Herb following that dreadful meeting:

Dear Herb,

I want to take a moment to let you know that I am very fond of you and that I fully appreciate all the care you have taken of me and that I am aware of how much you extended yourself on my behalf.

The reason I wished to make this change was based primarily on attitude. As brilliant and wonderful as you are as a doctor, so frequently you say things in such a way that really upset me. I guess our last conversation when you were so emphatic that it had to be the cancer somewhere else that caused the tumor marker to remain high upset me beyond measure. I hope you are not right—although you usually are. But you never leave me any reason to hope or feel positive. Over the last six months, each time I have seen you, you have reminded me that I will never be cured. I am fully aware of that fact—I don't need a constant doomsayer reminding me.

Again, thank you for all your wonderful care, and believe me, I do appreciate it.

Most fondly, Karen.

Karen wasn't bitter. She was determined, though, and to that end, we sought a new doctor who shared her determination. We chose Matt Lever, who was in Herb's oncology group, Beverly Hills Oncology Associates, and had covered for Herb several times when Herb was away lecturing at Yale or Stanford. Matt was a tall wise-man type, sensitive, kind, and, most of all, hopeful. When Karen had asked him the same question about her survival as she had Herb, the one to which Herb had answered, "There is no cure for you," Matt gave her hope by his very readiness to go to battle and destroy those liver tumors, to make them vanish. Matt was willing to talk details and progress.

We could have gone to UCLA or USC, but since Karen's records were at Cedars and because she had really sparked to Matt, I decided to go with him. Herb was incensed. "Let Matt take care of you, too," he snarled at me, firing me as his patient and slamming down the phone. If the two doctors hadn't been of equal stature, I'm sure Herb would have leaned on Matt to reject Karen's case, and to let her go to UCLA, or to hell, for that matter. But Matt insisted on rising to the challenge. I'm sure he got lots of grief from Herb, and I respected Matt all the more for doing what he did. Hell hath no fury like a world-class doctor scorned.

Matt set up the CT scan Karen and I had twice unsuccessfully importuned Greaves to do for us. The second time we visited Greaves was in mid May, six weeks after the liver surgery, and he had said that he would have to check with Herb as to the timing of the follow-up scan. I knew from my own field of surgery that it was up to Greaves, the surgeon, and no one else, to check on the results of his surgery and to order such a scan in a timely fashion. It was yet another clue to Greaves' ineptitude and lack of care.

I hoped the results of the scan would put Karen's mind at ease and give her the serenity she deserved. After the test, I spoke to Sanjay Shah, the radiologist. Usually cheerful, Shah was glum. I could smell bad news. There was residual cancer on the scan. It looked like a target, he said, a white border around a black center.

I didn't tell Karen. Instead I took her home to wait for the results, Shah, having promised to consult with a colleague, Roland Moody, who he said did more RFAs than any other doctor in the city. The early evening call confirmed the initial finding. This was on a Friday night. We couldn't reach Greaves all weekend. But I tried my best to buoy Karen up by accentuating the positive. "We got this much of the cancer, we'll get the rest. Two out of three lesions ain't bad," I said, doing my damnedest to be encouraging. Besides, I believed what I said. Medical science wasn't perfect by any means. If at first you don't succeed…The main point was to keep trying.

We weren't able to get an appointment with Greaves until the end of the following week. When we got to the office, his secretary made us spend half an hour filling out the same insurance forms she made us fill out every time we were there. "Procedure," she told us. Greaves wasn't any nicer. "What are you doing here?" he said, snarling as he walked into the room in his surgical garb, every inch the arrogant, God-playing stereotype of the surgeon. Not, "What's the matter?" or, "How can I help you?" We told him about the scan that had been sent to him, but that he obviously had not bothered to look at. "I'm sure it's just a hemangioma," he said, dismissing the unseen findings as an enlarged blood vessel. "She has a history of them," he said without ever looking at Karen, as if she were a specimen.

Finally, we went down the hallway into another room where he looked at the films. He pointed to the left liver lobe, where he had cut out the tumors. "There is no cancer here," he said. Then he pointed to the ominous black mass in the right lobe and declared, "Those radiologists have no idea what they're talking about. They're a bunch of jerks." I should have been relieved, but I wasn't. I was taken aback by his language, calling distinguished doctors names in front of his patient. We were not talking about a broken toaster, but a malignancy, a malicious, lethal, spiteful poison that played no favorites. What the hell was that dark black mass, that target? Why not go back in and get rid of it, RFA it? He was incensed at the suggestion. Even if it is cancer, he said, it was way too soon to RFA it again. "But it's not cancer," Greaves insisted, and, again, showed us the door.

In July, Karen's tumor marker shot up to eighty-nine. Her carcinoembryonic antigen, another cancer warning measure, was in the red-alert zone at 464. A CT scan revealed that the right liver lobe tumor, or whatever it was, had grown from five to seven centimeters, an ominous increase of 40 percent in one month. I called to make another appointment with Greaves, but he was away in Australia. His secretary was anything but helpful, making me feel like the doctor who cried wolf. "Dr. Greaves is fully aware of your wife's situation," she snapped. "He told you there was nothing to be concerned about." I wanted to strangle her with the phone cord.

Adding to the absurd horror of the unfolding situation, Karen found a lump in her right breast, or rather in the implant where her right breast had been. "It's just silicone," I said, having felt the tiny thickening. "The breast tissue is gone. You can't possibly get anything there." But Karen believed otherwise. To buy her some equanimity, we made an appointment to see the breast surgeon who had done her double mastectomy in 1999.

They say to always beware of any restaurant called "Mom's." I say beware of any doctor you see on television. It seemed as if I saw Armando Latini, her breast surgeon, on the news just about every week. He was always at big Hollywood charity events, auctioning Bentleys, giving away holidays in Bora Bora, posing with Elizabeth Taylor or Michael Jackson or Demi Moore. I suppose all this was in service of raising money to cure breast cancer, which is as noble a cause as there is, but I somehow preferred seeing the Saint of St. John's in scrubs rather than black tie. Yes, he was handsome and Italian and wore Armani suits and had a great singing voice, which he showed off doing a duet aria with Luciano Pavarotti at a charity function at the Hollywood Bowl. Yet I worried that this Bologna- and Harvard-trained doctor had become starstruck, and I wondered if he had time for "normal" patients.

I soon found out when Latini excised the new lump in Karen's supposedly non-existent breasts, it *was* cancer. Karen was right, as always. Latini believed that this cancer had spread there from the liver. The new news was so overwhelming that Karen barely reacted to it. My first thought was that Latini didn't "get" all the breast tissue when he did Karen's total double mastectomy. "The original breast cancer that had spread to the liver has now spread back to the breast," Latini said several times. Whatever was happening in her chest had nothing to do with his handiwork, Latini declared loudly. He seemed insulted that I had the audacity to raise the question. These were metastases from her liver. They were just Karen's awful luck. Cancer happens.

"It's metastatic liver cancer," Latini declared. "Nothing to do with the breast surgery. Niente."

To quell my own raging uncertainties, I asked Robin Levy, the famous USC pathologist I had met in the course of dealing with Karen's elusive HER2/neu protein, if he would take a look at the tissue samples from Karen's breast lump. Two years before, when I called every major cancer center from coast to coast, including the National Cancer Institute, Sloan Kettering in New York, University of California at San

Fransisco, and City of Hope, the one name that kept coming up was Robin Levy. Levy, who seemed to be on six continents every week, somehow found time to oblige me, but he returned with surprising news. The new breast lumps, he declared, were not liver metastases, as Latini had insisted, but breast cancer itself, breast cancer that had also spread to the liver. A big question arose: was Latini negligent of not having removed all the potentially cancerous breast tissue when he did Karen's mastectomy?

Whatever the answer to that question, the cancer was there, and could not be denied. This wasn't the moment for a lawsuit. There was no time for regret or remorse or revenge. The breast lump, tragic and unfair as it was, had been taken care of. The thing to do, in my mind, was to attack the cancer where it was now, in Karen's liver. Although I had had no luck piercing the impregnable fortress that was Greaves's front office, Matt Lever was able to get through. Unlike Greaves, Lever accepted the radiologist's report. It sure looked like cancer to him, especially with the markers going up the way they were. Matt scanned Karen head to toe and found no evidence of cancer except for the seven-centimeter growth in her liver. While Karen and I were sitting in his office, he reached Greaves in Sydney or the Great Barrier Reef or wherever he was, and told him he had to "go back in and RFA her again and be as aggressive as you can." Such a dynamic directive was highly unusual coming from an internist to a surgeon. Surgeons were usually the one to give such orders.

Things became even more surreal when we finally got to see Greaves a week later. To begin with, he kept us waiting in a large empty waiting room for more than two hours. No one else came in the entire time we were there, not even his secretary, Portia. No coffee, no apology, no nothing. According to what Portia told us later, when we arrived, Greaves was in with his lawyer. He's being sued for malpractice! was my first thought. When we saw him, Greaves looked tan and rested, as if he had been vacationing on the beaches in Australia, not lecturing in some dark classrooms. His line was the same: Karen didn't have liver cancer. What it was was just a hemangioma. Forget the numbers, the markers, the scans.

Still, I pressed him as to when he could go back in and re-RFA that right lesion. "Never," he said. "I don't do that procedure." But you just did it, I said. "I don't do that procedure," he said again. Case closed. I was mystified. Did he mean he didn't redo what he had already done on Karen? Did he mean that he didn't do RFAs through the skin, as opposed to cutting the patient open? Or that he did not do Radio Frequency Ablations at all, even though he had done it just three months ago? Or, worst of all, was he stonewalling and pretending Karen had never had the RFA to begin with? That would have been the stuff of horror films. In fact, Karen later said she felt like the Mia Farrow character in *Rosemary's Baby* when her fancy and stalwart Fifth Avenue doctor turns out to betray her and be a member of the Satan cult.

Tongue-tied at this turn of events, Karen and I asked Greaves if he could recommend us to someone else who did RFAs. He looked directly at Karen. "No. I can't refer you to anyone. How would it look, my making a referral based on my own failure?" I was stunned that Greaves could look Karen squarely in the face and say that to her. How could he have the audacity to sit there, a few feet from his patient, and, without any sympathy, kindness, or feeling, render such a pronouncement? This wasn't a failing grade on a test. Failure here meant an awful blow to Karen's life, her chance to live.

Of course, Greaves still did not believe that he had failed, or else he was bluffing. Whatever the truth, he was through with us, that much was clear. As we left, he threw us a parting shot. "Don't go to Ronald Moody. He'll RFA anyone who walks through the door. He's a total hack, and a quack. Don't go there." And he unleashed a spew of venom about Moody, about whom I knew nothing other than he was the RFA expert whom Sanjay Shah asked to look at Karen's first post-op scan that revealed the residual malignancy. Greaves also viciously attacked several other doctors whom he thought we might go to as backups, some I never heard of, some of whom were totally distinguished, extensively published, nationally known, and not worthy of his diatribe.

He also attacked hospitals, including Century City and St. John's. Greaves was out of control. He was obviously paranoid that he would be found out for his gross negligence with Karen. I wanted to call Thalians, the Cedars psych unit, and have him placed under observation. And to think he had been trusted with my wife's life!

This was my worst experience as a doctor with another doctor, and Karen's worst as a patient. This was way beyond *The Twilight Zone*. Yet Karen remained as determined as Joan of Arc going to battle. We immediately called Sanjay Shah, rather than Matt Lever. Sanjay was outside the Cedars loop. However fine a doctor and man Matt was, he was still a Cedars doctor and a Cedars man, and I seriously doubted that he would do anything to cross one of his esteemed colleagues, much less jeopardize his career, as I wanted to do. Here I was, a great medical practice in ashes, and here was Greaves, the Butcher of Bondi (Sydney's beach resort), ruining lives with impunity, if not high honors. But who was I, whose own career was in the dumpster, to blow the whistle on Greaves? I had no standing. So I tabled those thoughts. All that mattered was Karen, and Karen was in major jeopardy.

Naturally Sanjay sent us to Ronald Moody, the doctor Greaves had denounced so vehemently, but Greaves' warnings meant nothing at this point other than an indication of his fear of exposure. Moody was a shambling, relaxed, heavy-set man with a very kind face, the opposite of Greaves. A perfect gentleman, he steadfastly refused to criticize Greaves. However, he was equally steadfast in his belief that Karen's right lobe lesion was cancerous. He wanted to re-RFA it, and create safe margins around the lesion, something he noted that Greaves did not do.

Karen's new RFA, a five-and-a-half-hour procedure at Century City Hospital, went smoothly in mid-July 2002. It was carried out deep in the bowels of the hospital, four stories below ground. It felt like Los Alamos or Hiroshima down there, depending on your perspective. There were underground tunnels, a sickly yellow light, and no decorations whatsoever. For all the grimness, Karen was buoyed with hope. The doctors who we had gone to for help had taken away her hope, but there was an odd kind of hope there in this deep underground tunnel, a feeling of excitement. "I feel I'm in good medical hands at last, Alvie," she said.

After descending to the center of the earth, and signing a litany of those worst-case-scenario release forms, we were met by Ron Moody, who did his best to keep up the positive mood. Karen changed into one of those one-size-fits-no-one gowns, but I told her it looked like Dior on her. And then she went into Ron's nuclear chamber, lying down on the table in order for the magic rays of twenty-first-century RFA to destroy the cancer within her. Her anesthesiologist happened to be a guy I hadn't seen for twenty years, but a good guy nonetheless, the first doctor who did anesthesia for me in my new career in Los Angeles. He greeted me like a long-lost pal. I introduced him to Karen, assured her she was in great hands, and he put her under. "Say good-bye to cancer," I whispered to her. I hoped the angels heard me. Karen's last words were to Ron Moody. "Do a good job, please."

I retired to the adjacent room where a monitor and a scanner showed the progress of the procedure. I could see the long needle pierce Karen's skin and enter the liver. The needle would remain in place for at least ten minutes, the idea being to destroy a circumferential sphere of the cancer. Then the needle would be withdrawn and carefully directed into another portion of this sinister black mass. I had an eerie feeling sitting in this anteroom as the minutes turned into hours. It was deathly quiet, except for the rhythmic noise of the RFA machine. I watched as Karen's body, the body I loved, was punctured over and over, with holes burned into the flesh of her liver. Then a bell rang, and the procedure was over. Five and a half hours had gone by. Moody came out smiling. He was sure, as sure as one could be with unpredictable cancer, that the lesion was gone. That night I slept the sleep of angels in a chair next to Karen's bed.

Karen was discharged the next day, a lightning fast amount of time compared to the week of torture Greaves' RFA engendered. Alas, despite our reason to feel happy if not triumphant, we went home to a very sad house. Our beloved Ruddy Somali cat, Wojge, was dying of sinus cancer, bleeding and oozing pus from her nose. Just a year before, as Karen was starting her chemotherapy and her prognosis went from excellent to dismal, our other cat, the black and gray tabby, Doodle, died of lymphoma, my disease. Only Dexter, our indoor-outdoor cat, was going strong. That two of our "babies" had died of cancer seemed cruelly ironic. Cancer was plaguing. It had killed parents, it was killing cats, it was killing us. Wojge's distorted, swollen face reminded us of the cruel presence of the disease.

Karen seemed to forget her own travails when she saw Wojge, and she held her tenderly like the little daughter she was to us. Wojge had been with us all of our married life. The idea of her dying was too horrible to contemplate, but there it was. Because sinus cancer was one of my human specialties as a surgeon, I had done everything in my power to keep Wojge going, even finding a vet who would use the UCLA radiation equipment after hours to treat a pet with cancer. It cost a fortune, but, hey, this was our child. The vet became something of a friend to us. He knew all about RFA, all about Karen's illness, which he could discuss more intelligently, and more compassionately, than most people doctors. He sat us down and said what he was doing for Wojge was not a cure. We were in an end-game situation. I asked him how we would know when it was time to euthanize Wojge. "You will know," he said, calmly and sincerely. It was pretty spiritual, trusting our instincts for a moment we deemed unthinkable. But it seemed that moment was coming closer and closer.

Karen didn't have much time to care for Wojge. Just as I was congratulating myself on finally getting the right doctor, she began to be convulsed by waves of pain. At first I thought it was standard post-op distress, but after an hour, it got progressively worse. I annoyed Karen by initially refusing to take her to the ER. I told her we already had all the narcotic painkillers the hospital had, and that going there would only give us an endless wait among gunshot victims and sneezing and coughing people with highly contagious respiratory ailments. After being stabbed in the liver for five and a half hours, you're supposed to be in agony, I told her.

Karen got angry with me for not caring. She began crying, not in pique or sadness, but in real physical distress. "Please take me," she pleaded.

My poor wife; would anything ever go right for her again? Or was this some kind of infernal retribution for having had led such an ordered, exemplary existence, helping others and finding peace within for her first fifty-four years? I was still annoyed at having to go to the ER, which I saw as a waste of time. It would have been far better, I felt, to stay at home with our dying cat. Karen sensed my annoyance. Here I was, the great doctor, and even my wife wouldn't listen to me. We barely spoke en route to Century City.

Karen was admitted and placed on IV narcotics. I spent time talking to the kindly ER doctor who was friends with our new oncologist, Matt Lever. He told me how Matt had a famous father, who, after a brilliant career as a neurosurgeon, retired and began an entirely new career as a professor of astrophysics at MIT. Matt was brilliant, too, and had a stellar reputation, but he wasn't pushy or obsessive. I wasn't used to going to an ER as a patient, so it was an eye-opener to see how vulnerable Karen was, how much could go wrong, how valuable simple kindness and consideration could be, how scarce love was.

The next morning Ron Moody came in and gave Karen a CT scan, which showed her problem to be a major bile leak. Karen wasn't crying wolf at all. I was mortified that I had questioned her. The bile pouring out of her liver was as corrosive as battery acid, and it was getting all over her abdomen and pelvic organs. She quickly developed peritonitis, and the sleek stomach that she endured the most Draconian diet to maintain ballooned out as if she were nine months pregnant.

Cool and collected, Ron Moody inserted a bile drain. He didn't act sheepish or guilty for being at fault, for having done something wrong in his RFA that caused this disaster. That was because it wasn't Moody's fault, but rather Greaves's; it was Greaves who had left a defect in his sewing up Karen's liver capsule, which burst after this new procedure. I tried to make as light of it as I could with semi-conscious Karen. "The good news is that it's not another cancer," I told her. I joked about her writing a tour guide to the hospitals of LA, maybe even expanding it to include the fancy ones on the French Riviera, and in Switzerland, where the rich and famous go for secret procedures. Karen forced a smile, but it was a big effort.

Karen had seen her own father with a hugely distended abdomen when he was dying. I wondered if she was thinking of that now. But I never asked her. For all those setbacks, Karen was the most determined patient on earth. Nothing could make her lose her belief that this was a war that she would win, even if some of the battles didn't go as planned. One day at a time, I would tell her, but she didn't need to be told.

I myself could barely control my rage at Greaves, who had put Karen through this hell by not having done the original RFA correctly and for leaving her with a life-threatening defect. This was a classic case study in malpractice, but who had time for lawsuits? I had two sick and fragile loved ones on my hands, and I had to split my time between them. Through all her pain and despair, Karren insisted I go home and look after Wojge. So I did.

I found Wojge lying still on a chair, the fabric stained with blood and pus. At first I gasped, thinking she was gone. But when I scooped her up in my arms, I heard her purr-the sweetest sound I ever heard. I didn't dare stroke her head, for fear of causing her pain, but I held her gently, and then I made her a grande luxe feast of tuna and mixed seafood.

"*Ess, ess, mein kind,*" I exhorted her like a Jewish mother, and when she did eat, I beamed proudly ear to ear. If she had an appetite, she would live, I told myself with old wives' wisdom. It wasn't time. Not yet. I didn't know when. How would I know? A bolt of lightning? A burning bush? A voice from above? Whatever, I didn't want to hear it. I wanted Wojge, just as I wanted Karen, right here on earth.

My schedule involved giving Wojge my early mornings—feeding her, petting her, cleaning her wounds—then going to the hospital at nine to be with Karen until five, preventing life-threatening errors by the ever-changing, rarely up-to-speed cast of nurses. I would have dinner at home and stay with Wojge until eight, then return to the hospital and Karen until eleven. In a way I was glad I didn't have my practice, because I would have had to give it up anyway to care for my loved ones. Even on my hardest days of multiple surgeries, I was never so wiped out.

Late at night, I would talk to Wojge. She was one of the few living creatures that I could communicate with, share my deepest feelings, hopes, and fears with. Her green eyes expressed a care and concern over her Karen, just as Karen would ask about her. I found a lot of comfort in that little cat.

Moody's work was a veritable course in lifesaving. If only the hospital support staff had been as good as he was. We had to change rooms and floors four times in seven days, and there was no continuity of care in any location. The nurses would come in and start the Twenty Questions game: Why are you here? Tell me your history. What medications are you taking? What surgeries have you had? What are you allergic to? We were both developing an allergy to these repetitive interrogations. I complained, with all the courtesy I could muster, to nursing supervision, after the fourth move. The supervisor just hung up on me. How did she think a cancer patient felt? Not her problem, but it should have been. A patient's problem is a nurse's problem. It was no big surprise to me that just one year later this hospital went out of business.

The nurses seemed to change with every shift, so no one got to know Karen's medications or treatment regimen. Thus the bile drain failed to be flushed, causing a backup of corrosive fluid and a recurrence of excruciating symptoms. It required the patience of Job, which I did not have. Karen was always doing her best to temper my temper. After another awful week in the hospital, Karen pulled through and I took her home.

The worst part of Karen's homecoming was the night Wojge's time came. The cat was indeed happy to see her mommy, but the strength was ebbing out of her. I called the vet, and he said that she had lived far longer than he ever expected. He told me to contact "the other people," that is, the traveling vets who came to your house to euthanize your animal, the Jack Kevorkians of the pet world.

When Doodle died of non-Hodgkin's lymphoma, just two months after Karen's grim diagnosis of metastatic liver cancer, we had used these "other people." Then, as we had done with Tinker, we gave Doodle a proper burial in our garden in a casket we bought from the pet mortuary Animal Haven in Glendale. I reread the letter Karen had written to Doodle when she died. It seemed even more poignant now that all of our lives were becoming more precious with each passing day.

Dear Doodle,

Precious little Doodle. I will miss you terribly. I'm so sorry I took you for granted because I know you loved me and Daddy most of all. I know you were naughty because you loved us so much and were so possessive of us. When I look around the house and I don't see you, I feel such a terrible void. I especially miss you because I need you so much right now. Please forgive me if I ever slighted you. I didn't mean it, and please be a good in kitty heaven so you'll have friends to play with. And please look down on us and take care of us because we need you and your help so much right now. Daddy and I love you so much, and we will never forget you as long as we live. You were our very first baby. Dearest doodle, We'll love you forever and hopefully meet again someday.

All my love, Mommy

We sat there and wept as the traveling vet gave Wojge the lethal injection. I cried much more bitterly, for inside, I was praying to God not to take Karen from me as well. I held Karen close, kissed her tenderly, and did my best to deny the reality of her mortality. But what was reality? How long did Karen have? How long did I have? Wojge was actually given a year from her diagnosis, and she played by the rules, something I didn't want to do. I worried how our surviving cat, Dexter, (I refused to change the name, my fallen mentor notwithstanding) would respond to the loss of his last surviving "sister" when I saw Dexter sadly looking around the house for Wojge, meowing mournfully. "When will Dexter forget Wojge?" I asked the vet. "When you forget Wojge," the vet replied, and I knew exactly what he meant.

The decision to euthanize Wojge was much harder than actually coping with her being gone. Guilt, regret, sadness, and feelings of emptiness engulfed me. I imagined Dexter, Karen, and me "crossing the rainbow bridge" in the not too distant future. These were indeed morbid thoughts, but these were morbid times. Dexter was only thirteen and healthy. He might well be the one closing the drawbridge after the rest of us crossed over, it occurred to me many times. But I never shared these thoughts with Karen, nor did I ever discuss with her how she felt about the possibility of dying, about facing her final battle. I needed to allow her the conceit of an unlimited horizon, not a due date. Hope can be the greatest medicine. I needed hope, too, for Karen and for myself, hope and courage. I thought often of the courage Karen showed. Someone told us that courage is fear that has said its prayers, and that the test of courage is not to die but to live. I wanted her to live so much, as much as she did. I couldn't bear the thought of being without her, hence I wouldn't let that thought cross my mind. Denial, perhaps, but an essential survival skill.

In August we returned to Century City Hospital for a CT scan of Karen's abdomen. The good news was that Ron Moody's RFA was working; the site on the right lobe was healing, with no residual cancer or infection. But there was bad news as well: two tiny lesions had appeared next to the right lobe surgery site. Looking back over past scans revealed that the seeds of these growths had begun to sprout right after Greaves' surgery in April, but they were so small then, and nobody noticed. Now they did. My worst paranoia had been realized. Greaves' wedge that he cut into the cancer had indeed caused it to spread. Karen's prophetic words came true.

I had to break the bad news to Karen in our garden on a perfect August night filled with fireflies and the smells of the flowers and the soft summer breeze. I first told her the good news, that the infection was gone, then downplayed the bad by saying the radiologist wasn't sure, but these "tiny dots" may be small cancers, but that Ron Moody could zap them in nothing flat. I tried to be a combo of Knute Rockne, Billy Graham, and Tony Robbins when giving Karen a pep talk, plus I did some Emeril Lagasse as well, exhorting her to suspend her ideals and mainline some animal protein in the interest of energy. You can never be too rich or too thin, I told her, but you can also never be too strong and too vital. I'm not sure she bought any of it, though she did begin nibbling at ribs I would buy her from Gelson's luxury supermarket.

When Karen was discharged from the hospital, we noted that she developed a fever of 100 to 101 every evening around six o'clock. There were no obvious precipitating symptoms. The fever seemed to resolve with Tylenol, only to reoccur the next evening. This went on for months. Because Karen's fever would still not go away, I began calling everyone I could to find its etiology and a cure. One person I spoke to was the Cedars radiologist who had been present when Greaves had done his botched RFA in April. I introduced myself as Dr. Reiter, Karen's husband, and said I wanted to know more about RFA and its possible relationship to Karen's persistent fever. After a brief conversation, this very sincere woman seemed to forget she was speaking to the husband of the patient, or, as I sensed, she felt compelled to express her feelings toward Greaves.

This radiologist volunteered, against all canons of medical ethics and confidentiality, that Graves had no idea how to do RFAs and had previously referred all patients who needed the procedure to someone else. Why Greaves was experimenting with Karen, the radiologist had no clue. The doctor also mentioned that Greaves had spent one hour doing the RFA on Karen, the same procedure that took Moody five-

and-a-half hours. This conversation was very strange and disturbing, for sure.

Ever since Karen's diagnosis, I had been speaking to the National Cancer Institute in Bethesda, Maryland, where billions of dollars were funneled for research and treatment every year since President Nixon began the heralded War on Cancer thirty-five years earlier, although the cure still remains elusive. I had a conversation with institute doctors about Karen's fever with several medical experts in RFA. They confirmed that a five-centimeter lesion, the size of the cancer in Karen's liver, typically takes a minimum of four to five hours, not Greaves' one-hour express version.

It made me feel betrayed again, and furious that Greaves was allowed to be practicing medicine. Life was unfair, to be sure. Death, which Greaves had brought to Karen's door, was more unfair. This was way beyond malpractice, I thought.

I went on to call three more of the experts at the NCI who knew me and Karen's case by this point. Each asked me to go over in detail every step of the Greaves story. Each doctor noted that the target shape that Greaves had dismissed as a benign hemangioma was classic for cancer. Each doctor noted that the RFA involving this lesion takes a minimum of four to five hours. And when I related the surgery date—April 15, 2002—and then the scan date—May 31, 2002—they interrupted me and asked, "What did the first scan show?" I replied, "The scan on May 31 showed…" They cut me off again. "No, Dr. Reiter. What did the first scan show, the one done right after the RFA?" My heart sank to its lowest depth. They were referring to the scan that each insisted had to be done immediately after the RFA, the scan Greaves adamantly refused to do, the scan that might have prevented the hell Karen was going through.

Each time I heard that phrase "immediately after the procedure" my heart sank. I knew I had been right, but, in Karen's case, my being right and her being well were two different matters. I had trusted the wrong man, a bad man. It all showed that no matter how much research I had done, and how many references I had gotten, and how meticulous I thought I was, things could still go terribly wrong.

Speaking of wrong men, Karen now discovered still another breast lump where Latini supposedly had gotten all her breast tissue. This time, it was in the left breast. I didn't dare blame it on silicone again, nor did I dare think of returning to Latini. Instead we found a highly regarded female breast surgeon, Dr. Lucille Ward, who removed the lump in an outpatient procedure. It was cancer again.

In the course of switching to Doctor Ward, I had called Latini's office to request the surgeon's operative notes on Karen's double mastectomy. The office couldn't find any, nor could Blue Cross when I went to them as backup. To my amazement, the records didn't exist. Latini had never billed Blue Cross, our insurance provider, for this very expensive five-and-a-half hour surgery, which surely would have been worth $20,000. But why not? Further investigation revealed that Latini had made no surgical records or surgical reports on Karen. In medicine, the first thing you learn is that you must document *everything*. According to the canons of ethics and all medical law, if it's not written up, it didn't happen. When confronted with this major oversight, Latini blithely offered to dictate some notes now, three years after the event. How could he possibly remember?

This missing, or never done record nightmare continued. I asked to see the records of Karen's last two visits to Greaves's office: the first, when he had so unprofessionally lashed out at "those jerks" the radiologists, and the second, when he declared that he did not do RFA (after having done it on Karen). "I'm sorry, Dr. Reiter," we were told, "we can't find any records."

And what about St. John's, this 800-bed hospital that purports to be one of the leading institutions in California? The law required detailed records of all operations. The hospital did not note the absence of a five-and-a-half-hour cancer surgery operative report? No doctor anywhere is allowed to continue on staff without completing and signing all his records, especially the operative reports. What was not revealed that made the surgeon and the hospital forego payment, I wondered? The surgery also included an insertion of breast tissue expanders by the plastic surgeon, Dabney Lee, which took about half an hour. Why was there no record for that? And how did the anesthesiologist bill for a five-and-a-half-hour surgery without an operative note—or did she?

Maybe Italian medical training dispenses with written surgical reports, but I don't think so. The bottom line is that there was no record to research to see what kind of job was actually done. Even Herb's office didn't have a record of Latini's work. How could Karen's own oncologist, who needed to see those records before outlining a course of chemo, not have them either? If I were to believe the world-renowned pathologist Levy, and I did, Latini had done a horrible job, a potentially fatal job. Here were world-class doctors practicing world-class negligence.

When Karen first discovered her breast lump and after Latini's supposedly lifesaving double mastectomy, she was given a 95 percent chance of survival. After Greaves' butchery had spread the cancer that Latini's butchery had left to fester, those chances, which had diminished to 5 percent, were declining fast. To me 5 percent was better than nothing. Karen deserved every chance in the world. Now she had almost none.

What could I do? After my experiences with Larry Carmen, the idea of a lawsuit was anathema. I had knowledge, but here was a case in which knowledge was not power, not by any means. However, I wasn't the aggrieved party. Karen was. "I tried my best. These doctors let me down," she said, over and over, as if unable to believe that they had. We were both outraged that these doctors had played with her life, committing the grossest of negligence. If my career could be destroyed over some petty billing issues on procedures whose quality no one ever questioned, then Greaves and Latini, who had put Karen at death's door, should both go to the electric chair, not to mention Herb, who, by giving her Tamoxifen, might have headed all of this off entirely. Call it sour grapes, call it husbandly protection, call it an eye for an eye, but don't call it good medicine, whatever you do.

I wanted to shield Karen from lawyers, but she wanted to take action. She felt severe wrong had been done, and was almost biblical in her sense of justice. Accordingly, I called four top malpractice lawyers whom I had known about as a doctor as the last guys you'd ever want to be going up against in court. Then they were "the enemy," but now I wanted them on my side. I presented Karen's case to them. Great case, terrible plaintiff was the identical reply of each of them. If medicine was cruel, the law was even crueler. As a metastatic cancer patient, the odds against Karen were long and bad. None of the lawyers was willing to gamble that Karen would survive long enough to get to trial. The opposition would see to that, dragging out discovery and depositions for years.

None of the lawyers believed Karen had years. Months were more likely. They weren't trying to hurt my feelings; they were just quoting the charts and bailing out. They'd rather have a fool for a client than a corpse for a plaintiff. One of the lawyers spent close to two hours on the phone talking to me and Karen. He was a board-certified doctor as well as an attorney and was one of the most formidable lawyers in the country. He was appalled at the care Karen had received, and I knew just from his tone of voice and his choice words that he felt Karen's pain. In an attempt to assuage her anguish, he recommended that she think of this cancer as taking its natural course—and not as the fault of these doctors, even though he knew it was. "You become less hurt," he said, "venting your anger at God and this disease, instead of at some mortal."

Those were odd words indeed from a litigator, but there they were, and Karen did accept them, especially when she saw the hopelessness of getting a top gun to go to court for her. As the lawyers told me, the only way they could get past a judge to a jury, who they conceded would love Karen and her situation, would be if Karen's chances of survival were better than 50 percent, which they were not. Otherwise, a bad doctor could be drunk, on drugs, totally negligent, severely harm the patient, and still get off scot-free. Life, and law, couldn't be more unfair. Sick people and old people, it seemed, were not entitled to equal justice, or any justice, in our supposedly wonderful democratic system.

I had never been more depressed in the entire course of Karen's illness. Those actuarial charts rarely lied. I'd wake up in a cold sweat with the horrible realization that, according to those charts, in which nothing was certain save death and taxes, my wife would be gone from me by this time next year. For the first time in our fight against cancer, I got the sinking feeling that I was in a losing battle.

Matt Lever wanted to put Karen back on chemo. Matt, unlike Herb, was a fighter, and he didn't adopt the watch-and-wait attitude in Karen's case. Xeloda was his drug of choice, an oral regimen that obviated the need to travel to the chemo chamber and did not cause the hair loss that can depress a patient almost as much as the prospect of dying. I was game for the drug, but I felt Karen needed a break from the endless hell of bad medicine she had been going through. Accordingly, I asked Matt if I could take her on a trip. People in the Renaissance always traveled with their doctors, as anything could go wrong. So Karen, a Renaissance woman herself, would be traveling with her doctor. Matt, to our delight, said yes. The only question then was where we would go.

Our first choice, under normal circumstances, would have been Europe. Spain in September would have been perfect, a place of history and culture where Karen could speak and savor the language. But it was too far. Argentina was another possibility, but it was even farther, and besides, Eva Peron had died of cancer. That would surely come up. I wanted cancer, death, all bad associations out of the picture. I hated that word "cancer." I sat alone for several nights thinking where I could take my love on what I think I knew might be our last voyage, but which I totally censored in my active thoughts. I wanted so much to believe that she would survive for another round of treatment, then another, and another…Neither of us could accept the idea of impending death.

Yes, I was a doctor, and I knew the odds, but I was also a husband, and a human being, with frailties and fears and hopes and dreams. Science and reason often clashed with spirit and passion. I thought I understood the dying patient before. As a doctor, I had dealt with death and dying, but nothing in my career had prepared me for the profound complexity of the mental and physical process of a severe illness like Karen's, nor with the nightmare of dealing with a medical system that was simply not compassionate. Conflict and turmoil roiled within me.

I never asked Karen if she thought this was our final journey together. I didn't dare, and she never said a word, as if it would be bad luck. We just lived day to day. I did try to pump her up about the upcoming chemo, and I talked about new vaccines in development somewhere over the rainbow. There were hard facts, too. Dear Mimi made it to eighty with breast cancer. At fifty-four Karen had twenty-six years to go. Maybe it was the New Math, but I'd try anything to keep things hopeful.

Finally we decided to go to Northern California, from Eureka to Mendocino to San Francisco, the redwood forests and the deep sea waters, "This land was made for you and me," as Woody Guthrie sang. We had some of the world's greatest scenery right in our own backyard, so why not go for it. Neither of us had ever been up north, so it would be an adventure. Matt Lever gave us his blessing. Chemo could wait. And we were off.

Karen was a little anxious at first, wondering if she was strong enough to go on a long trip. I assured her she was, and she trusted me. We flew to the lumber barony of Eureka and rented a car. The town's name, Greek for "I have found it!" revealed its Gold Rush origins. Eureka is one of California's best-kept secrets. Bordered on one side by spectacular Humboldt Bay, the other side is surrounded by mountains lush with redwoods, a reminder of the area's rich logging heritage. There are beautiful old Victorian homes, high cliffs, crashing waves, and a harbor busy with fishing boats.

We stood on cliffs overlooking the sea and watched the waves caressing the shoreline, powerful but not destructive. Change the language and a few signposts and this could have been the rugged coast of Spain, a Norwegian fjord, or the coast of Cornwall in England, which we had visited in healthier, happier days. We were restricted in our vision only by our imaginations. Karen smiled and looked so peaceful, with the salt-laden breeze gently caressing her face and tossing her hair. Whether shrouded in mist or bathed in dazzling in sunshine, the shoreline gave us the occasion to enjoy, to reflect, and to hope, a total contrast to the ugliness of the cancer invading Karen's body. It was all nature, a nature that could be so bountiful, and yet so cruel.

There were also dramatic sand dunes in this nature preserve. One morning we went walking in those pristine, rolling dunes amidst seals, pelicans, herons, and mosquitoes. This was the time of the big scare about the West Nile Virus, which never really materialized. Still, when I noticed a mosquito perched on Karen's delicate white chin, I had to decide what to do. "What are you staring at?" she asked me, oblivious to the insect on her face. I told her there was a mosquito on her face, and she began to scream, "Kill it! Kill it!" So I did, with a gentle slap. Too gentle, it turned out, because within moments her chin began to swell with the effects of a mosquito bite. She pulled a mirror out of her pocketbook. "How could you let that happen?" she cried. "I'm going to die of West Nile Virus." She was serious, which I took as a healthy sign of her will to live. Here she had metastatic cancer, and she was much more concerned about a very rare, unlikely, and hypothetical affliction.

Things got even worse when we noticed a large sign at the entrance to the dunes, which we had completely missed before. It read something like, "Caution. This area is closed. Beware of insects, especially mosquitoes. If you are bitten call your doctor immediately. By order of the Humboldt County Department of Health." I tried to make a joke about it. "Well, darling, you won't have to worry about cancer any more." She was not amused. For the next week of our wonderful last trip, Karen spent an inordinate time in front of the mirror watching the bite get redder, taking her temperature, waiting to go into a West Nile seizure. It took a whole week before she could declare herself West Nile free.

I did my best to distract her with a lot of driving through the Victorian gingerbread palaces of Ferndale, the rolling dairy farms, the towering redwoods. I would have been happy to settle here, stop time, disease, aging, chemo, tumor markers, probation, community service, all of it, just stay here and grow plants and milk cows. When dinosaurs roamed the earth, a tree grew that we now call the redwood. These majestic trees, which used to cover much of the area but were now an endangered species, still gave us hope. They are the tallest living things on earth, growing to heights of 350 feet and beyond. To the lumber companies, the redwoods were a bonanza, immense logs of straight, beautiful, long-lasting timber. What nature could not bring down, man could, cutting, in a few decades, huge stands of trees that had taken centuries to grow. What we saw were the survivors, and they gave us a sense of life, of survival. Was Matt Lever to be our own Smokey the Bear, to put out the fire of cancer? Was Matt to be Karen's John Muir, the California naturalist who saved much of the state's natural beauty? Would Matt save my natural beauty, Karen? We hoped so.

Our voyage continued down the dramatic, dreamy California coastline to Mendocino, the fuchsia (bleeding heart) capital of the world. In Mendocino we witnessed one of the most remarkable coasts in the world, eaten away by the ocean into the most singular and fantastic shapes. We stayed at an inn with a certified organic garden and farm, a farm with animals and only vegetarian fare. Karen was right at home. It was just what this doctor ordered. It was hard to believe that we were here with cancer, and it was very difficult to rid my mind of that dreadful word. We were in the midst of everything Karen loved: gentle friendly farm animals, cats everywhere, and beautiful gardens filled with flowers of all colors, shapes, and fragrances, spread with the onshore sea breezes and a full course of vegetarian foods. If only they could provide a cure.

A few more days in the urban oasis of San Francisco eased us back to the reality of Los Angeles, if not the chemotherapy. Matt was his usual optimistic, high-spirited self and started Karen on Xeloda, the new oral chemo. He did another scan and found no new lesions and no growth in the new tiny ones. Like shooting ducks in a barrel, I tried to reassure Karen. If she could survive West Nile, those goosebumps would be easy to vanquish. Karen would take the Xeloda, and, almost like a prayer, say, "Come on, pills, do your work."

They did, but only to a certain degree. Her tumor markers began coming down from sixty, but never got to that magic under-thirty safety zone. Then Karen started to develop reddish lesions on the sun-exposed parts of her body, which I feared were possible skin metastases. I called the drug's manufacturer, Roche, in Nutley, New Jersey, and asked their scientists if this was a drug-related manifestation. They were flummoxed; they didn't know.

I took Karen to a dermatologist, who was puzzled. He said the lesions looked like a sun-related pre-cancerous condition after being treated with 5FU, which she was not taking. That's it, I said. Her chemo, Xeloda, was a form of 5FU. So this chemo was killing precancerous skin lesions before they were visible. This was the only silver lining to the cloud of chemo we could find.

I called the drug company back and filled out papers for them documenting my finding, of which they were not aware, so it could be immortalized in the drug's package insert on side effects. One of the researchers told me, "Your wife is amazingly fortunate to have you as her advocate. What you are doing is remarkable." The pat on the back felt good in the lonely, isolated life I was living. The time when I was fully involved in my practice seemed like lifetime ago.

In return for an improved tumor marker, there is always a price with chemo. Karen's price was developing something awful called hand-foot syndrome, in which raw, excruciating lesions formed on her palms and soles, the corrosiveness was so destructive to the skin that it could completely obliterate fingerprints. I had to put greasy ointment all over her hands and feet to moisturize the skin. Just walking and using her hands became an ordeal. Drastic diversion was in order. My solution was to find Karen two new cats to keep our sole survivor, Dexter, company.

Our obsession with cats, I liked to remind myself as to not seem too oddly obsessive, was not without historical precedent. Although there are ten million more cats in this country than dogs, cats have not traditionally been universally admired. Ambivalence toward them dates back to the dawn of civilization. Some early cultures venerated cats as benevolent deities, while others believed them to be agents of the devil. Over the last 7,000 years, the cat has evolved from a wildcat to a lap cat. The ancient Egyptians loved cats, mummified them with the pharaohs, and made them sacred religious symbols. The Greeks and Romans were far less sentimental, but did value their cats' rodent killing prowess. The later Christians didn't like cats a bit, however. During the Inquisition, Pope Innocent VIII declared owning, or even feeding, a stray cat a form of witchcraft punishable by burning at the stake. The stray cats were burned, too. In any case, the Christians finally calmed down (Muslims were always pro-feline because of the prophet Mohammed's great fondness for the animals), and brought cats to the new world where they thrived and prospered, first as rat killers and later as man's real best friend. Theophile Gautier noted that "God created the cat to give man the pleasure of caressing the tiger." Leonardo da Vinci said, "The smallest feline is a masterpiece." Karen and I could not have agreed more.

The death of our beloved Wojge left us without our great companion. We visited multiple animal shelters looking for a replacement. Karen took great pleasure in the task; it fortified her and made her smile. We finally found a female calico kitten with beguilingly languid green eyes, and then a handsome black and white tabby male. Both had been slated for euthanasia. Ours was a feline *Schindler's List*. We wanted to save them all.

We named the girl Beanie and the boy Cecil, cartoon characters of forty years ago. In the comics, Beanie was a little boy in a beanie cap, and Cecil was a seasick sea serpent. In Bel Air, we indulged in a little gender bending. Additionally, I became Captain Huff 'n Puff and Karen was a ship called the Leaking Lena. I assured Karen in October when we adopted these two kittens that even though she was leaking, she would not sink. I, the great captain, along with Beanie and Cecil, would keep her afloat. Those dear cats would soon become the one saving grace in the darkest days of our life that lay directly ahead.

After countless treatments

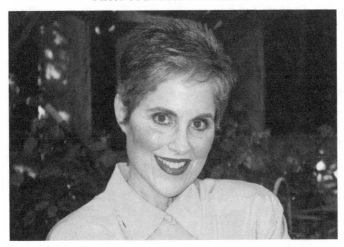

Still fighting

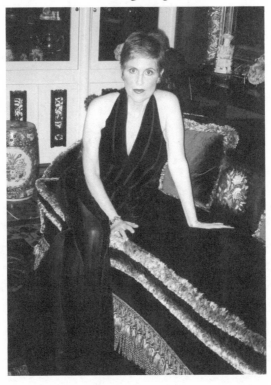

Chapter Eleven

NEVER SAY DIE

At some point in the fall of 2002 I noticed the word "palliative" on Karen's bulging medical folder. Before the word had been "curative." Cure means just that: end the disease, go and live your life. It means that you and medicine have won the battle.

In a system where winning is everything, palliative care is the poor stepchild. It's an admission that the patient is at the end of the line, so let's make her remaining time as pleasant as we can, provide the best quality of life we can, lessen the pain, ease her into the inevitable. It is a combination of active and compassionate therapies intended to comfort and support the patient. But the omission of hope, the hope implicit in the word "cure," is a knife in the heart. It means the person is going to die, not as we all are, at some later date, but in the foreseeable future. It meant that medicine was writing my wife off. That sat terribly with me, and I just couldn't accept it.

I never had been a throw-in-the-towel sort of doctor, but rather a tenacious fighter who could not accept defeat. A case study in my doggedness in giving a bad risk a great effort came early in my career in LA in the person of Rafael Proenza. Rafael Proenza was a sixtyish Hispanic auto shop worker who presented to me with a huge neck mass that was metastatic cancer from his larynx. It was a hard, immobile, golf ball sized protrusion that fortunately, if there was any fortune to be had here, had not spread further into his body. I presented his case to the tumor board at Cedars.

After making a thorough presentation of his disease and its extent, I proceeded to lay out my plan of action, i.e., the surgery I was going to perform. After listening politely, the assemblage of experts who evaluated most cases at the hospital advised radiation only; not for cure but to palliate his symptoms because they believed his cancer to be incurable. These doctors believed that even with radiation, Mr. Proenza would be dead in six months. I, on the other hand, had taken to heart my teacher Paul Donald's dictum that every chance to save a life must be taken. I wanted to do a combined therapy in search of a cure with a laryngectomy to remove the original cancer and a radical neck dissection to remove the lymph glands to which the cancer had spread, then follow both procedures with radiation to eliminate any remaining cancer.

Due to the advanced stage of the cancer, the patient developed a blockage of his airway and required an emergency tracheostomy. This emergency surgery then caused the need for further therapy for the cancer because, once you cut across the tumor field, it theoretically can spread, thus necessitating immediate treatment. I then deferred to the tumor board's decision to treat the patient with radiation therapy, even though I did not believe that this was the correct course. He underwent a full course of radiation, but since this was not a curative measure, and since I still believed that I could cure the patient, I decided to take him to another hospital and do the surgery that I wanted to do in the first place. I advised the family of the pros and cons and let them make the final decision. I guess I was persuasive, because they gave me the thumbs-up to proceed. So I enlisted the aid of another "never say die'er" and scheduled Mr. Proenza for admission to the French Hospital in downtown LA, actually in Chinatown, which a hundred years before had had a sizeable French community, which was the hospital's original raison d'etre. He was admitted six weeks later, the appropriate time after completion of the radiation treatments. I felt as if I were a medical Scarlet Pimpernel saving my patient from the gallows of Cedars.

We did a successful surgery through the skin that had been inflamed by the radiation treatments. Unfortunately, the patient developed a complication, not an unexpected risk, because the radiation had caused extreme destruction of the tissue and the wounds dehisced and a fistula, or tract, developed between his throat and skin. This meant that when the man swallowed, some of his food and saliva would seep out from his throat onto the skin of his neck. This proved to be a source of severe anxiety and discouragement for him and his family. Maybe I had gone too far. Maybe we should have listened to Cedars and settled for palliation.

I waited for the wound to close, but it did not, so I had to take him back to surgery. I feared that the cancer had returned and was what was causing the wound problems. Visibly, there was no evidence of the cancer and this was borne out by negative biopsy results, no evidence of disease— "NED" as Greaves had arrogantly and mendaciously hissed at me.

Rafael was now cancer free, but he didn't care. I tried to encourage him to eat as much as possible in spite of the spillage he was experiencing from the wound. Noticing that he was losing a lot of weight, I began to monitor the input and output feeding charts. Every day, trays of soft food were brought to him and though on paper he appeared to be maintaining proper nutrition, his appearance certainly belied the charts.

One evening when I went to visit him, I noticed his dinner tray sitting, almost completely full, with nothing having been eaten. When I questioned the food worker about the daily intake of my patient, she informed me this was the norm on her shift and that the patient was really not eating anything at all.

The conundrum was resolved! The nurses were not paying attention to what he was eating and simply indicated that the patient had consumed whatever had been served to him without any consideration for what he had actually consumed, or in this case, not consumed.

After that, I contacted the family and was told that the patient was in severe depression and did not want to live. I could understand his despair and frustration, but for my own part, having worked so hard and so long to save his life, I was not about to let him starve himself to death. I took this poor skeleton of a man, now down to eighty-five pounds, and shook him. "You don't have cancer any more and you will not die on my shift!" I shouted at the poor fellow, scaring him terribly. I'm not sure how much of my attitude was Hippocratic, how much bravado, how much ego. I surely didn't want that pompous Tumor Board to win. They were wrong, dead wrong. My combined approach gave Rafael at least a 40–50 percent chance of long-term survival, if not a cure.

I then made nightly visits to the hospital and spoon-fed him myself for several months. I was rewarded by seeing him regain much of his lost weight as well as a new desire to live. He eventually left the hospital. We had won the battle against the demon cancer. I was glad I had been inculcated by such a strict taskmaster and had developed the tenaciousness needed to deal with patients with advanced cancer such as this. He was alive and fifteen years post-op, coming to see me for an office visit for an unrelated problem. I wept with joy about how healthy and happy he was. If I could do this for my patient, how could I do any less for my wife?

Little things, however, caused me some despair. Karen was growing weaker, almost imperceptibly, but the grind was taking its toll. Her tumor marker numbers would never make it into the safety zone of "normal." It was like being back at Bronx Science, trying to crack a certain level on the SATs and falling a few points short. Close, but no cigar. Forget Harvard.

I knew Karen was in trouble when she tossed out her treasured cache of *Prevention Magazine*, *Weight Watchers Magazine*, and other health magazines. She had stopped reading them, and they were just piling up. But then she went back out to the garbage and fished them all out and arranged them as perfectly as a librarian. I breathed a sigh of relief, at least for now. She was now eating ribs and ice cream, which I brought her to shore up her strength sapped by the powerful chemo drug Xeloda. For all this indulgence, she still wasn't gaining weight, which couldn't help but alarm me. Karen never commented on her dietary changes, her fall from purity and grace, and I never teased her about it. It was no laughing matter.

During this time, I thought about the mice that Sylvan Minsky had been experimenting with in an effort to a develop a cell line of pure human metastatic breast cancer for future experiments that could eventually help to find a cure. Minsky had called me several months earlier. "Are you sitting?" he asked. With that introduction to the conversation, I didn't know what to say, so I sat down immediately.

"They came into my lab and destroyed all the mice," he said. "I don't know if your wife's was among them."

"Who destroyed the mice?" I asked.

"The mice police," he said.

As it turned out, it was a team of people including veterinarians assigned by the Research Study Committee and various other bureaucratic officials. Minsky had set up Karen's liver cells to transplant into the mice to develop these xenografts and did it as quickly as possible.

"I was trying to save Karen's life, and I knew time was of the essence." he said. Because he had set up the experiment so quickly, he had not followed all of UCLA's stringent bureaucratic rules to the letter. Minsky related that the type of approval needed for this could take many, many months, a time frame Karen could not afford.

Minsky told me that the chances of success for this particular cell line without the development of a mouse mutation were less than one in ten thousand, and to date, the scientific community had little success. But his work, in the early stages, appeared successful.

They stripped Minsky of all his laboratory privileges. It seemed so drastic and pointless. Here he was trying to do something worthwhile, to save lives, and the UCLA bureaucrats were behaving like the Nazi book burners in World War II. No Nobel, no vaccine, no cure, no hope. One more loss, one more step down the staircase to oblivion.

After the initial letdown, I decided not to give up. Minsky had told me to call the Medical School Dean's office. At first, I thought that was ridiculous and impossible. Talk about bureaucracy. But I tried after he gave me the telephone number.

Minsky had an excellent reputation as a researcher, as I would find out, and he had written many papers on breast cancer. So I summoned my wits and courage and called. The dean was not in but I could talk to the head of pathology, who, by coincidence, was the dean's relative.

Minsky warned me about this fellow's lack of care and concern and derisively referred to the dean as Hollywood dean—in reference to a huge Hollywood donor to the medical school and the person for whom the School of Medicine is named. The pathologist talked to me briefly about the fact that protocol was not followed and if—IF—this experiment was resumed, it would take many committees and a long time for approval.

I thought of Karen's expected life span at this point and said something to the pathologist, who promptly and rudely hung up on me. I called back immediately, numbed by his brazen attitude; his secretary told me that the phone connection had been interrupted and he wanted to continue our conversation but that he just left—all in less than two minutes. So much for the Hippocratic oath on his part!

I asked his secretary who else I could speak to. She gave me the name of another medical school dean. I was fortunate, this dean was in and was very cordial, but not very helpful. Finally, I told him, "Dean, my wife is very sick with cancer, metastatic cancer. We need help." He told me we could try contacting the university's chancellor, who was also the head of animal and human experimentation. I almost began to cry. I profusely thanked the dean, who at least cared and didn't give me, or by association, Karen, short shrift.

The next day was a holiday so I waited to call, thinking all the time of those mice carrying Karen's cancer for future experiments. Even though I had hope, I had doubts in my heart about where this would lead. Mice, cancer experiments, vaccines, a cure for Karen? Did Semmelweis, Marie Curie, Albert Einstein, or Jonas Salk start this way? I also thought I would have a better chance reaching the governor of California or Laura Bush in the White House than the chancellor of UCLA.

Maybe not undaunted, but definitely driven at this point, I called his office and reached his secretary. She told me, after listening to my story, to e-mail his office. Karen was sitting beside me by the phone. I yelled, "I don't know how to e-mail. Please, please help."

Karen tried to calm me. "Don't argue with them, Alvie," she said. I almost cried. What grace she had. But before I could make a next move, the chancellor himself got on the phone.

"What can I do for you?" he asked, in the most understanding tone.

I said, "It's a long story."

"I have time," he said. "Tell me your story."

I proceeded to tell the story of Karen's history from the breast biopsy on. He took an hour of his precious time to listen intently to the whole sorry mess. "I'll see what I can do," he said.

As good as his word, he rang back three days later.

"I found three mice," he announced proudly. "We'll take care of this." The chancellor promised to get Minsky back on track.

"That's a good sign," Karen said with a big smile, and I prayed her reading of the runes was as prescient as it usually was.

Karen's birthday was December 8, the day after Pearl Harbor. She was going to be fifty-five. By chance, one of her closest friends, Betty, was going to be married on that day and was planning a fabulous party. We decided to go. We rarely went to black tie events, and, although Karen loved looking nice in clothes, she rarely dressed up. Aside from charity events, the Oscars, and the Emmys, LA isn't a black tie sort of place. Because of back problems, Karen was uncomfortable wearing high heels, but she decided to grin and bear it, so off to Nordstrom's we went to shop for the upcoming occasion. A friend of another friend was a salesgirl in the gown department. She knew of Karen's illness and was very kind to us, pulling out countless gowns in the finest silks and satins. "You look so great in green," the salesgirl said. "Do I?" Karen responded sadly. She knew the future was short, but to please me, she tried on dress after dress, finally choosing a flowing black silk number that was very Manhattan.

Next came the shoes. She chose a pair of black velvet pumps, trying to justify the expense by promising to wear the outfit on New Year's Eve as well. I worried that she might stumble in the heels, but she breezed around in those magic shoes as if she were a model on a runway. The wedding, in the Grand Ballroom of the Four Seasons Hotel in Beverly Hills, was everything we thought it would be, with champagne, caviar, flowers galore, a full orchestra, and the most dashing crowd. I told Karen all these black tie revelers were really here to celebrate her birthday. The wedding was just a cover.

The bride stopped the festivities to raise a birthday toast to Karen, and all eyes turned on her. She was the most beautiful, radiant woman in a sea of distaff beauty. What a dramatic change from the horrible isolation she had endured ever since her cancer diagnosis in 1999. This was like her coming out party. I was buoyed with hopefulness, but then I thought about the cancer and its odds and nearly dissolved in tragic tears during the enchanted evening. How could Karen be leaving a world so bright and gay? One minute your loved one is alive. And the next she is dead, no longer sitting across from you, toasting you with champagne, holding you on the dance floor, filling your heart with joy just with her dazzling smile. The evening was wonderful, and yet it was grotesque at the same time.

New Year's Eve was equally conflicted for me. The party, which we were attending with some doctor friends, was at the Regency Club, an elegant English-style lair of tycoons owned by super tycoon David Murdoch, whose fortune was based in part on Dole Pineapples. As she was dressing up, Karen said, "Alvie, I think this is the last time I will be wearing high heels." Her words gave me an unbearable heartache.

I put on a great performance and kept a smiling façade. I joked that we would still have parties to suffer through in her upcoming recovery stage. "If you think these heels are bad," I teased, "think about the new chemo regimes you'll be going through, and the experimental vaccines. Being a survivor is no piece of cake."

An unkind cut that befell us at the beginning of 2003 was the early retirement of oncologist Matt Lever, who decided he couldn't take the pressured rat race of Los Angeles anymore. He married his new girlfriend and was going to move to a ranch in the Napa Valley. Karen took it with a brave face. She really liked Matt because of his kind, never-say-die tenacity. She bought him a beautiful crystal horse as a going away present and sent him a note on our behalf: "To our favorite 'City Slicker.'"

Dear Matt,

We, like all your other patients, are devastated that you are leaving. You are a wonderful person, compassionate, caring, and charismatic—not to mention tall, dark, and handsome! We will miss you terribly and feel cheated we only had your exceptional care for such a short time. However, we do wish you and your bride the best of luck on your new adventure and agree that you are probably wise to be doing it while you still have your sanity.

All our love, Karen and Alvin Reiter

P.S. Can we please contact you with any questions as to treatment?

Once Matt moved, his oncology office, the one he shared with my erstwhile savior, Herb Bloomfield, refused to give us his new Napa number. "Respect his privacy!" the secretary said. Luckily, Matt was listed in Directory Assistance, and, of course, he took our calls.

Matt's replacement was a distinguished, WASPy oncologist named Guy Hill, who, amazingly enough, had been Karen's father's oncologist back in 1988. Unfortunately, he had no interest in saving lives, or at least Karen's life. Just as Matt was leaving, Karen had a very dispiriting bone scan that revealed that multiple lesions had reappeared on her spine. We had lots of questions, lots of anxiety. Guy Hill had lots of patients, his and Matt's, and he was two hours late for our first appointment. He arrived in a huff and cursorily glanced over Karen's thick chart, which he, or any doctor, should have done long before the actual appointment. Our immediate impression was that he didn't even care to find out what she was dying from. His mind may have been on his last patient, or his next patient, but it wasn't on Karen.

It wasn't as if Karen had acne or heartburn; she had metastatic cancer, and she deserved all his attention. She got fifteen minutes. There was no preamble, no how's your family, no nothing. Hill was sweating. He seemed shaky, nervous, not the reassuring, take-charge man he had the reputation of being. He seemed even more nervous as he examined Karen and palpated her enlarged, hard liver, a finding consistent with widespread cancer. In fact, her cancer seemed to freak him out. He should have known exactly at what stage it was and all of the treatment options at that stage. He didn't. He was totally unprepared and that did nothing to inspire the confidence Karen, or any patient, desperately needed. Hill's ability to break bad news was also abysmal. But his failure was Karen's loss and Karen's pain and heartache. I tried to be concise.

I just have four questions, I said to Hill. "The first is about the Xeloda chemo drug that is sickening Karen." He cut me off. "I don't have time for this," he snapped. He wouldn't spare her a second. He just dumped her. Karen, more vulnerable than ever, broke down crying. She rarely cried, so I knew this was the epitome of cruelty, reminiscent of the sadistic Greaves. Hill's response to Karen's tears was to leave. Karen may have been a lost cause, but Guy Hill had no right to make her feel like one. This man was the Terminator of Cedars, a cruel, cold machine who didn't even promise, "I'll be back."

Once we finally tracked down Matt in Napa and told him of the Hill fiasco, he admitted that he would have recommended another colleague, Dick Helfenstein, who was young but very kind, which seemed to be the prime criterion in choosing a doctor at this point, but that he had chosen the older, more experienced Hill because his history with Karen's father should have engendered compassion, if not nostalgia. We changed doctors and were happy to be getting a "good guy." Our Nobel Prize fantasies were over. I accepted that we weren't going to find a miracle cure for Karen. I just wanted to keep her alive, with me, as long as possible. I wanted years, not months; I wanted to beat the actuaries. She had been put through all this awful, incompetent surgery, and for what? She might have done far better, lived far longer, without a stitch of it. But I couldn't look back. I seized every moment and treasured having her frail body by my side.

In late February, 2003, things took the dreaded turn for the worse. In the last weeks of January, Karen, tiny, skinny Karen, had been gaining weight. At first I congratulated myself that my junk food diet for her was making her more robust and stronger. But then Karen began measuring her waist, which grew from a svelte twenty-eight inches to forty-four, almost a foot and a half. It was something called ascites, an accumulation of fluid in her abdomen from her diseased liver. And then the pain started, slowly building up to something as bad as when her liver capsule leaked acid all over her viscera.

I knew we might be in big trouble, but I was still in denial that the end was upon us. I was hoping that Karen's problems were caused by the toxic Xeloda, which I had read (I read endlessly) could cause hepatitis. By this time, the liver enzymes were rising and Karen's beautiful eyes were now tinged with yellow as a result of the elevated bilirubin that comes with liver disease. Maybe if we would stop the Xeloda, her abdomen would subside and she would live happily ever after…at least she would live. So I got on the phone again after reading journal articles about Xeloda by doctors from MD Anderson Cancer Center in Texas.

I continued to be amazed at the time, courtesy, and consideration the doctors there gave to me. I remembered my phone calls after Karen's diagnosis of metastatic liver cancer, and how much time the doctors from leading national institutions spent with me. The only time these conversations ended was when I hung up the phone.

After a careful discussion of the timeline of the illness and the medications, the doctors at MD Anderson rejected my theory about hepatitis, since hepatitis would have initially appeared when she started the medications, not now.

I had a call from a doctor at the National Cancer Institute in Bethesda, and he asked that I take her to Bethesda. "We will take care of her," he said. I would have taken her to Lourdes for holy water if I thought it would help. I was very impressed by this kind and unsolicited offer from this caring NCI doctor.

I soon received a call from my doctor-friend at Sloan-Kettering in New York. I told him about Karen's case again, including the swollen ascites-filled abdomen and jaundiced eyes, and he said, with loving care, in the most compassionate but firm voice, "Alvin, forget the poisons, the chemotherapy, the radiation filled CAT scans and MRIs. Karen needs some quality of life. Focus on the time left. Forget the cures. I had been seeing the letters QOL for all the years of Karen's illnesses as well as my own, and the meaning of those letters had never before hit home.

I spoke to Dick Helfenstein, who sent Karen to Cedars for a scan of the abdomen. Afterward, he called and told me, out of Karen's hearing, that, according to the radiologist, Karen's liver had basically exploded. Then, worst of all, he concluded, "Bring her in. Your wife is dying." I did ask Dick one big favor, which was to partly blame Karen's swollen stomach on the Xeloda and hepatitis rather than the cancer. And Dick obliged me, telling her what I asked, with the addendum that "There may be some cancer there as well." Part of my caregiving was softening the blows.

"Your wife is dying." It was the first time anyone had ever spoken those direct words, and though I knew it, the actual words felt like a sword through my heart. I immediately had a flashback to *Love Story*, when the doctor told Ryan O'Neal those same words, "Your wife is dying." The scene acted out for celluloid at Mt. Sinai Hospital in New York, ironically, the same place where I did some of my surgery training a year later. And in the end of the movie Ali McGraw did die. The end was near if not here. Nevertheless, I still couldn't accept it. I'm not sure, but I think Karen may have finally begun to accept what I could not. I think her exploding waist demoralized this eternal Weight Watcher so much that she seemed to accept it as one of her Signs from Above. She didn't want visitors; she didn't want to see her friends, maybe because she was ashamed of being so bloated, but more likely because she wanted to rest in peace, as it were.

If only she could have. We opted for a new kind of combination chemotherapy that had shown some success with breast cancer, but Dick had reservations about it because of the excruciating side effects. Karen insisted on it, though, saying she could take it. After being admitted to Cedars, she was placed on the intravenous medication, which had to be accompanied by heavy sedation and a morphine drip for the pain.

Dick had thoughtfully ordered physical therapy to make Karen more comfortable and to help mobilize her body to prevent stasis of blood in her legs, which would prevent blood clots that had the potential to go to the brain, heart, or lungs. When the physical therapist came the first time, Karen was very sleepy and she asked him to come back later. Karen, polite as ever under all circumstances, didn't want to be a pest.

The next day he returned. Seeing that Karen was still somewhat sedated, he left the room and told me that if she refused his treatment one more time, he would not return, as if visiting Karen for two to three minutes to check on her condition was a great effort on his work load. I asked him, instead of walking her down the hospital corridor, to please passively move her arms and legs to prevent blood clots and make her, with mild physical stimulation, feel better. It seemed like a sensible request, but the therapist refused.

"She doesn't want to have therapy," he said. "It's not on her chart that she's incompetent to make decisions." He spoke without any sense of humanity or care.

This hospital to the stars was a living hell. I snapped, but rather than waste my breath on this incompetent ignoramus, I ran to find the Director of Nursing. I went from building to building, flush with anger, sorrow, frustration, and a deep sense of shame—shame for the entire medical system that had lost a good part of its humanity.

I regained my composure and found the Director of Nursing. "If you continue to let my wife wallow in her urine and feces, I'm going to throw her over my shoulder and carry her out of this hospital," I said simply.

The startled nurse bid me to sit down. I then proceeded to tell her about Karen's condition and the lack of care she had been subjected to, which included a nursing staff that basically ignored her. This was a throwback to the 1960s when patients who were in the end-of-life stage were placed far from the nursing station and the medical personnel, or perhaps it's not a throwback but a situation and attitude that still remains quite prevalent in our medical system, a system that is broken, I thought. This same system prompted Dr. Kübler-Ross to write her classic *Death and Dying* around 1965, a book that remains pertinent today. I guess you have to shout to be heard. The nurse promised us instant results and extended a profuse apology.

When I returned to Karen's room, I found her in tears. "Dr. Helfenstein came by while you were gone. He says I have to go home. There's nothing more they can do for me," she said, groggily, through the painkillers, in more emotional pain than I had ever seen her. Another massive SPIKE violation, breaking awful news to Karen without me there, the one person who could have softened the blow. I was appalled. How could Dick, my source of hope, betray us like the others?

Before I could call Dick to find out what his discharge talk was all about, the hospice doctor came into the room. It was like a bad stage play, an inept *Waiting for Godot*. Hospice had arrived with the idea of making Karen's final days, months, whatever, as comfortable as possible. Here was palliative care in person. Insurance only pays for six months of hospice. My first thought was they had given Karen six months to live. At that point, I would have leapt at six months.

The hospice doctor was another matter. He looked just like Death in Bergman's *The Seventh Seal*, and he scared the hell out of me. He had piercing eyes in a long, thin, sunken face ending in thin, colorless lips and a grey, pointed goatee. All he needed was a black robe and scythe. He came over to the bed, stuck his long, bony finger into Karen's swollen beach ball of an abdomen and said, "I've never seen anyone recover from that." No attempt at empathy, no I'm sorry, just a long finger with a long face. And then he left.

Karen, numbed by painkillers but still conscious, heard this and was speechless. It was insult added to the injury of Dick abandoning her. Abandoned to this? Was Karen's response acceptance, or sheer terror? I don't know. But when Death walked back in to claim Karen as his own, I made one of my snap decisions and sent him packing.

I then called Dick, who didn't return my urgent message for what seemed like hours. When, finally, he did call, he said he had tried looking for me before he spoke to Karen, and I jumped down his throat for breaking such terrible news to her all by herself, afraid, sick, weak. "I'll give Karen what she wants," he said. "If there's a chance, let's take it." Dick put Karen back on chemo. We had to give life one last shot; I had seen the alternative and didn't like it.

I thought about Elizabeth Kubler Ross's five stages of dying. First, the denial, "not me." Second, the anger at this uninvited illness; third, the bargaining for time, usually with God; fourth, the depression about leaving your loved ones and at how they will cope; and finally, a spiritual acceptance of the impending death, making peace.

Karen was not ready—or was she?—for the Final Curtain, Stage 5.

I wasn't about to turn her room into a morgue. I brought in plants but no flowers, as there is an alteration in the sense of smell during chemotherapy, so a rose may smell like an onion or vice versa. A friend brought balloons of different colors, sizes, and shapes, which seemed almost to fill the room. I obtained multiple bulletin boards with the help of the hospital maintenance crew and pinned up exciting travel posters and pictures of our trips together, as well as photos of our friends and their notes of hope and support.

I also brought in the cats, one by one, because, if anything could prolong Karen's stay on this earth, it was her love of these wondrous creatures. I knew that no pets were allowed, so how did I get them in? The hospital had guards at the entrances, and although I wasn't a terrorist, I had to be clever and cautious. I had a cat carrier and put Miss Beanie the calico kitten in it and told her not to meow. The security guard looked at me menacingly and said, "No pets are allowed in the hospital," literally blocking the entrance. Thinking quickly, I thought, and almost stammered, "I'm Dr. Reiter, and I'm doing cat experiments in the lab."

"Right this way, Doctor," the guard said.

Up in Karen's room, I unloaded the dish for food and the litter box I had brought in the day before. I took some new Science Diet out of the closet and filled the small bowl. I was hiding them under Karen's bed so no one would notice when the charge nurse came in.

"You know, Dr. Reiter, and you should know better, no pets are allowed in a patient's room."

"But these are our little children," I pleaded, like a child who had been caught doing something naughty but nice.

"I don't see anything," the nurse responded with a knowing wink and left us alone.

Out came Beanie from her personal pet carrier. But Beanie was shy and hid under the bed. Eventually I took Beanie home because the hospital frightened her. Karen however, was overjoyed to see the kitten, even though most of the time she was under the bed instead of on top of it.

The next day, I brought Cecil, again through the Homeland Security defense perimeter. When Cecil, a playful, black and white tabby, came out of his carrier, he immediately jumped onto the bed and curled up at Karen's feet, giving her lots of love but lots of space as well. Cecil must have been a doctor in one of his previous nine lives. He was right at home in Karen's room overlooking the towering palms and mansions of Beverly Hills, a perfect fantasy world where there was no disease, where everyone was skinny and perfect and lived happily ever after. Most of the stars and moguls who created this myth did come right here to Cedars to die, but somehow, the myth of eternal sunshine was stronger than the reality of decay, suffering, and death.

One day, in the hospital hallway I ran into Carlton Starr, who first observed Karen's tiny breast cancer in 1999. We had been out of touch with Starr since then.

"How's Karen?" he asked in all innocence, with a warm smile underlying his truly caring tone.

"She's dying," I said.

"What happened?" he asked.

His face continued to show concerned interest until I related the findings of the spread of cancer to the liver. When I got to the part about Michael Greaves and the RFA, Starr blanched. He turned white as a ghost.

"He should not be doing that procedure; he doesn't know how to do it. He's at the low end of the learning curve." He was visibly moved to the point of tears at Karen's condition. Starr's voice trailed off. The tears started to fall. Doctors rarely cry, so this was some commentary on the bright and vibrant patient Starr had thought would live to a hundred. Now he saw how wrong he was.

And then he hugged me, which isn't doctorly either. But it was the mark of a real man.

Week after miserable week went by. Karen was unable to have a bowel movement, an observation it seemed only I had made. A basic part of hospital record keeping is to note the patient's intake and output, what they are eating and drinking, and what is being eliminated by the kidneys and bowels. When I spoke to some of the nurses taking direct care of Karen, they had no idea she had not moved her bowels in weeks.

I suggested to these nurses and then to our doctors to try stool softeners, laxatives, or even an enema if it was safe. "That's a good idea," they said, a phrase I would be hearing again and again after my multiple observations and suggestions, a phrase which eventually frustrated me. The hospital then tried these bowel-stimulating measures, but nothing worked.

Some of the nurses were awful and uncaring. Most were devoted and compassionate but were caught up in this tragic conflict between an ever-increasing patient workload and decreasing nursing staff and wages. There was no continuity, which is vital to a patient's well-being, not to mention avoidance of deadly error. There seemed to be an entirely different cast of characters every shift and every day. Where, I wondered, did these nurses go? Were they on a conveyor belt that went from one hospital to another around the world? Were they phantoms? Were they all illegal aliens, on the run from the IRS? Cedars was a virtual United Nations of nursing, with people from every country, some of whom spoke very little English. There was no such thing as forming a "relationship" with a nurse or aide. And even if you did find a nurse you connected with, you would only be disappointed when you never saw him or her again. At the same time Karen's bowels were not moving, neither was her appetite. She ate little and had to be given supplementary nutrition. Yet she hung on for dear life. My only concern was how long she could endure the pain, starvation, and deformity.

Fortunately Karen's friend from childhood, Valerie Stewart, came by to visit, as she had been doing since Karen had fallen ill. (It was Valerie's twin sister's wedding we had gone to on Karen's birthday.) Valerie strongly suggested that we get sitters to stay with Karen in the room, a suggestion that turned out to be a blessing and a necessity. This corp of women became indispensable caregivers, helping Karen get to the bathroom, ambulate, and eat, as well as provide companionship and shore up the nursing care. Why, I wondered, didn't the hospital suggest this earlier? Why didn't I think of it myself?

And then something totally unexpected occurred. It was late March, in Karen's third week at Cedars, the day George W. Bush invaded Iraq. Out of nowhere, Karen had a bowel movement, a massive bowel movement, engendering true "shock and awe" at the bedpan station. After this breakthrough, her intestines and peristalsis went back to their normal function. Dick Helfenstein rushed over and ordered an abdominal X-ray, which showed no blockage and normal function. Soon Karen was up and walking and her bloated belly subsided greatly. In addition, her tumor marker and liver enzymes went way down.

"A miracle has happened," Dick told Karen. "You are doing better than anyone on the whole floor. I'm so pleased." Dick stroked Karen's head. She looked up at him with a weak smile. Dick was proud of her, proud of himself for staying the course. That's how patients can make you feel. It's one of the true joys of medicine, healing, helping, winning the battle against disease.

Now that Karen had become a "winner," the attitude of the hospital seemed to change overnight. The physical therapist who had wanted to write Karen off as a basket case suddenly leapt at every chance to be with her and give her therapy. One day he waltzed her down the corridor, Fred leading Ginger in fancy footwork. All the nurses began smiling, springing to attention, asking about the cats. "They're home, waiting for their mommy," Karen would tell them, her eyes alive again. No more Rainbow Bridge, I quietly prayed. Good-bye palliation, hello cure.

A week later, Karen was discharged, walking out of Cedars all on her own, nearly a new woman. In your face, Death, I said to myself. I got into our car and tried not to look back but ahead to some quality time with the woman I loved. I wanted life, not end of life. Maybe Karen was ready and I was not, but that bright springtime California sun shining on Karen's beautiful face lulled me under the ether of the Hollywood dream of life everlasting, as opposed to the top-dollar medical hell we were leaving behind. We were so happy to be coming home alive. No one offered us any specific instructions in regard to pain management, diet, activities, or how to deal with going home after this horrendous confrontation with near death. Cedars' highly vaunted pain management team never appeared either during the hospitalization or upon discharge. There was no visit from a social worker, therapist, or home health care aide service. As far as I know, there really was no cancer support service at this hospital. No real effort was made toward Karen's well-being. There was a definite lack of clarity on their part as to palliative, end-of-life, and hospice care. No one was offering any information, and we didn't want to stick around the charnel house of Cedars to wait for it.

I assumed I would continue with the sitters at home and basically take care of many things myself. For some time I had to make choices about my role in Karen's care, as physicians have long been discouraged from providing medical care for their own family.

The main change in the house was the hospital bed I ordered for our upstairs bedroom. The antique bed where we slept was far too high for Karen to get in and out of easily. I also got Karen a shower chair, where she could sit while being bathed, and a walker, to make getting around more stable when necessary. I hated to see her as a semi-invalid, but I loved just seeing her, so that was the price I had to pay.

Once we got back home, Karen resumed chemotherapy on an outpatient basis, this time with an intravenous drug called Navelbine, another pleasant sounding medication with the usual brutal side effects. Back to the infusion room, the chemo lounge, the roller coaster of hope and despair. Still, as doctors say, where there's life and an open flowing vein, there is hope, and hope is what kept us going through all the rest.

One day after her first treatment, Karen's abdominal pain began again. This time the pain was much more intense. She was sent home with some morphine "lollipops." I had a whole medicine cabinet of other painkillers from previous hospitalizations and procedures, but I had no idea which might work for her and which were contraindicated given her delicate condition. Dick Helfenstein was away for the weekend (why do problems always arise on weekends?), and the covering oncologist said just give Karen the lollipops, up to five lollipops per hour. I had already given her two and, because morphine and other narcotics are respiratory depressants, I was reluctant to just keep dosing her like that.

That afternoon I was all alone with Karen at home. Even with all my medical training, I felt completely helpless watching her writhe in glassy eyed pain, and I was discouraged by the oncologist covering for Dick. It seemed he had no experience in pain management even though he certainly should have—or perhaps he didn't care. Did he write terminal cancer patients off or was it just take-two-aspirin-and-call-me-in-the-morning attitude? I opened the medicine cabinet again and stared at the tiny brown bottles of oxycodone, hydroxycodone, codeine, percodan—all filled with promises of relief yet carrying with them the risk of respiratory death. So I went back to giving Karen the flavored lollipops, and eventually, after hours and hours of intense suffering, the intense pain subsided.

Once Karen's pain subsided, I was able to leave her with the sitter to run my caregiver errands. I was able to go to my lymphoma support group on the following Tuesday evening. When I shared my recent experience with Kathleen, the oncology social worker who ran the group, she hit the roof, at me and and at Cedars. Cedars has a big pain management team, she told me. She couldn't believe we didn't consult together before Karen was discharged. I had no idea the team existed. No one had mentioned it to us.

Nor had I any idea how the law had changed. Regulation of controlled substances had led to fear of prosecution. If you gave the patient pain medication, you had to justify it, because of the fear of addiction. "Treating cancer pain may lead to dependence," Kathleen told me, "but not addiction. Ten years ago," she continued, "if a doctor gave a patient narcotics for cancer pain, he could lose his license." How many people suffered because of that ignorant baseless fear, I thought.

Today, under the Intractable Pain Treatment Act, physicians are not subject to discipline for prescribing controlled substances in treating intractable pain, defined as a pain state in which the cause of pain cannot be removed or otherwise treated. If a doctor didn't give narcotics today, he could get into legal trouble. The law had come full circle and pain management was a major deal. At first the doctor could go to jail for prescribing narcotics to cancer patients, and ten years later he could go to jail for NOT prescribing narcotics.

After group, Kathleen took me to her office and showed me reams of books, brochures, pamphlets, all written, not for medical professionals, but for patients and their families. "Pain Control: A Guide for People with Cancer and their Families," American Cancer Society; "Cancer Pain Treatment Guidelines for Patients," American Cancer Society; "Breakthrough Cancer Pain: Questions and Answers for People with Cancer and their Families," American Cancer Society; "Controlling Cancer Pain: What You Need to Know to get Relief," Cancer Care; "Understanding Chemotherapy: A Guide for Patients and Families," American Cancer Society; and many more covering many aspects of cancer care in readable language. There is even a Web site: www.cancernetwork.com.

Then she showed me even more stuff on hospice care. "Why," she despaired again, "didn't Cedars sit you and Karen down with a team of doctors, nurses, social workers, psychiatrists, rabbis, whatever, and prepare for this moment, which was bound to arrive? No one should ever wish for death because of the reluctance of a practitioner to provide the most appropriate pain medication."

I was traumatized by Kathleen's well-meaning rant. Why indeed didn't Cedars counsel us, or at least give us some of this material and urge us to read it? If UCLA had it, why didn't Cedars? Cedars should have sat me down before Karen's discharge and at least skimmed the surface of pain and bowel movement home care. But they didn't. Palliative care, it seemed, was second-class care, or in our case, no care at all. Maybe, I agonized, it was because I had insulted the hospice man, Dr. Death. Maybe this was his territory, the empire of terminal pain and suffering. But then I reflected that this wasn't the case. Cedars was simply careless, if not uncaring. Not everyone accepts hospice. Some just want a hospital, a hospital that does its job.

Reflecting upon Karen's painful ordeal of a few days earlier, I learned even more. Even though established guidelines for pain management have been published, 80 percent of patients initially seen in palliative consultation have been subjected to dosing errors. The most common error is failure to give round-the-clock opioids. Ongoing pain is best managed by taking pain medication on a schedule and at regular intervals. Most people usually take medication in response to specific pain, and when the pain goes away they stop taking the medication. This is not an effective way to manage ongoing pain. They should not wait until the pain returns or gets really bad.

Pain can surge—called breakthrough pain—and additional medications that act quickly can address this pain. If the pain is allowed to persist and escape, it may be more difficult to control, and with higher doses, depressed levels of consciousness, depression, nausea, and other toxicities develop.

Kathleen told me that Karen should have had a pain patch delivering dosage around the clock, which would have helped her avoid many painful experiences. This patch is easily applied to the skin and can be easily changed by any family caregiver.

I told Dick Helfenstein about the horrible pain she had suffered, the ineffective lollipops, the literature I found at UCLA and *not* at Cedars and then suggested a pain patch this time around. He was very thoughtful and said, "Good idea." In fact, he had said "good idea" to just about everything I would suggest. At the hospital, I had suggested giving Karen a blood transfusion to make the chemo more effective. "Good idea," he had agreed, and indeed her pallor lifted and she felt better. I had suggested giving Karen iron and vitamins. "Good idea," he said. I suggested a pain patch to anticipate the agony and short circuit it before it could really kick in. "Good idea." But why didn't Dick think of all that? I recalled a California case in 1998 in which a family sued, claiming that the doctor engaged in elder abuse by neglecting to effectively treat the pain of an eighty-five-year-old at the end of life. The family won $1.5 million. I thought of the Carly Simon song, "I Haven't Got Time for the Pain" and shuddered in despair at the system I was in.

At this point, Karen's pain was controlled by the pain patch, but she had become constipated. I read up on the new chemo and discovered that a potential side effect was that it could slow peristalsis and cause constipation. But she needed the chemo, so what could we do? Fortunately, the solution did not involve life-threatening respiratory depressants. Karen had consumed as many fluids as possible, continued her Weight Watcher habits, including high fiber foods such as prune juice. But to no avail. She had taken the laxative route along with stool softeners but no results. I called the oncologist to see if an enema would be safe in respect to the abdominal cancer. The oncologist on call cleared this but showed no sympathy to my reluctance to administer the enema myself. Her attitude was cold and totally indifferent, sadly typical of many members of our profession. Ironically, she was the one to whom I had first suggested giving Karen a transfusion to make Karen feel less fatigue, less depressed, and to help the effectiveness of the chemotherapy, all things I learned at National Cancer conferences. She refused, stating the transfusion would only last a month. Talk about end-of-life care. At first I flat out refused. Even though I had spent my life doing major surgeries, there was something about giving my wife an enema I couldn't deal with. My first instinct was that I didn't want to hurt her. That someone else would have hurt her less was totally illogical, but where was logic at this stage of a crazy game? It was a border I didn't want to cross. I insisted on getting a visiting nurse, but after numerous calls, I saw that none were available for at least twelve hours. "Oh, Alvin, please, just do it," Karen begged me. She reminded me I was a doctor. "You can do anything," she said. So I did. And it worked. But it was anything but easy.

For the next three weeks, Karen held her own. Friends would come by for visits, which was a welcome change from just the three of us— me, Karen and the sitter, six if we counted Dexter, Beanie, and Cecil. I was amazed at their skill in providing Karen with a diversion, a chance for at least some pleasant thoughts, if that was at all possible.

Each Friday we would go to Cedars for outpatient chemotherapy. I thought we would have at least a year together, maybe more. But by the fourth Friday, Karen's abdomen began to swell again, and the day after her weekly chemotherapy, she began throwing up, which she had never done before. I watched helplessly as her frail, swollen little body heaved and choked. It was awful. She broke an antique glass all over the floor in the bathroom. That was the glass she had used for years to brush her teeth. Now it was shattered in a million pieces. Karen didn't even cry. She was too weak. She was defeated. Every time I thought my heart couldn't break any more, it did.

Because Karen needed fluids, I called Dick Helfenstein, who sent a nurse over to administer an IV. This was the beginning of the end. All my hopes, and Karen's, that she had pulled off a miracle, were dashed to the ground. We both knew she was dying this time. That Saturday I wanted to get out of the house just for an hour or so, just for my own sanity, but Karen begged me not to leave her, not for a second.

"Please, Alvie, please. Stay with me." At that point I knew it was all over. My strong brave wonder woman was now a frightened, quivering little kitten, in total terror of the unknown that was staring her hard in her beautiful but stricken face. My impression was that she thought she would die at any minute; these were indeed the desperate hours.

I would have taken Karen to the hospital, but Dick was away again for a few days, and I didn't want a stranger, or worse, Guy Hill, looking after Karen. Karen and I didn't speak about death. It was the Great Unspoken. Karen barely talked at all. She just lay there in that awful shroud of fear, clutching my hand, staring sadly into space, reminding me of my mother in her last years.

"Rub my feet, please, Alvie," she asked me. I was happy to give her any comfort whatsoever. It was a sign of life, and, to me, anything that spoke of life was a pleasure in this miasma of death that was about to engulf us. As I touched her, I tried to savor every sensation, every moment, the glory of her tender skin, the skin of a baby, because I knew

347

that in a few more days, I would never be able to touch her again. Ashes to ashes, dust to dust. Those awful words were becoming so real.

I thought about keeping Karen at home to die among her cats, her flowers, her antiques, her books. It used to be that most people who died of non-acute causes died at home. That was the tradition. A hundred years ago physicians had little to offer beyond the easing of symptoms associated with disease. By the mid-twentieth century, the growth of science and industry brought about sweeping changes including sanitation, improvement of working and living conditions, and lifesaving and life-prolonging treatments, and the focus was shifted from easing suffering to curing disease. In our own times, death is equated with medical failure.

Institutions have replaced the home as the most common place where death occurs, and in this setting, the caregiver has changed from family to strangers. All that was anathema to me. I was a humanist. As a scientist I embraced progress, but as a person I embraced love, and love was something I hadn't seen at the hospital. Yet I had no choice but to surrender to the inevitable.

When Dick returned, I arranged to take Karen to the hospital. Dick had me call to make a date for the next morning with the paramedics, who wanted to take her to UCLA, which was the nearest hospital, but then agreed to take her to Cedars, to her treating doctor.

That night, unable to sleep, I sat up until 3 a.m. talking to the very kind sitter, who came up with a question I couldn't answer.

"Dr. Reiter, how are you going to get Karen downstairs?"

I hadn't thought of this at all, but the sitter made me realize that the stairs were too narrow for a gurney. "Do you have a small chair that might make it?" she asked.

I spent the rest of the predawn hours locating the right vehicle, a dirty foldable lawn chair that I had to wash. When the paramedics arrived, we wrapped Karen up in sheets. I watched in tears as the paramedics carried my love down the stairs and into the ambulance. It was biblical, wrapping her in swaddling clothes and laying her in a manger. Except she was leaving the world, not coming in. Karen's helplessness was pitiful. I couldn't stop crying, knowing when we closed the door, Karen would never come back into our home, the home she loved so much. The three cats stood by like a feline honor guard as the door to the ambulance slammed shut. Farewell, my lovely.

One of the paramedics was Israeli and Karen somehow had a weak chat with him about her summer on a kibbutz as a teenager. I sat in that bumpy little ambulance with her, holding her hand, trying to be strong, wanting to give my life for hers. Oh hell, I thought, then she'd be as lonely and miserable as I was going to be. When we got to Cedars, it wasn't as if Karen's bed of angels was waiting for us. We couldn't be admitted directly to a room. Protocol demanded all entries be through the Emergency Room, which was in particular bedlam that day, screaming people with gaping wounds, dreadful flus, bloody car wreck casualties.

Dick did come down and got us a tiny anteroom to house Karen, lying on her gurney, until a room became available. "I want out, I want out," Karen mumbled to him. I don't think she meant the little anteroom. I think she meant this so-called life of hers. "I want out," she said again. "Don't worry," I assured her, grasping her hand. "He'll snow you," I whispered, which she knew meant he'll put you under morphine to kill the pain—a euphemism for something else? I prayed.

Dick started her on IV morphine right away. An orderly came in and tried to insert a Foley catheter to collect Karen's urine. He had no

349

idea what he was doing. Tears of pain fell from Karen's haunted eyes. I pulled him aside and practically begged him to get someone more senior. I could have done it myself, but, as with the enema, there was the dignity of our last moments of marriage together that I was trying to preserve. A new orderly came in, did the job, and left us alone to sit in teary silence with each other.

I remember the pet story where our kittens in heaven were waiting at the Rainbow Bridge for Karen so they could all cross over together. But I wasn't a Rainbow Bridge guy at the time, much as I was touched by it. I couldn't do bridge talk. I just sat there and held her hand and stroked her forehead and mourned.

Eight hours later we were admitted to a room on the so-called cancer floor, the same floor where Karen's mother had died. Karen had insisted on a different floor the last time we were in Cedars in February, and as sick as she was, she insisted on a different floor now. But there wasn't a bed available elsewhere, and this was the cancer floor, so the best we could do was put her on another wing, which had been redecorated since Mimi's passing.

By eleven that night Karen was out of it, and so was I. I took a cab home to feed the cats and collapse. I had no dreams. I was too tired, I guess, or maybe I was in subconscious denial. I was back the next morning, terrified of finding Karen gone, but there she was, asleep like a baby. I was thrilled that she was still alive, but then I thought about it, and realized that mine was an impossible dream. She wasn't going to wake up, come back, be her fabulous self, live. It was all over. I was so conflicted, so pained. I wanted Karen—and me—out of our misery.

Dick Helfenstein came and outlined his plan of action, which was to gradually increase the morphine drip from 10 mg to 20 to 30 until…He didn't say that level would kill her, but as a doctor I knew about morphine, and I didn't say no. Karen was comatose at this point. Yet somehow, as Dick and I were talking, she began waving her hands, with her eyes closed, crying, "Help me, help me, help me." Dick took her hand, said, "It's Doctor H. I'm here to help," and eventually she stopped crying out.

"Karen is not at all in an awake or semi-awake state," Dick said. So I took her cry as a plaintive plea from the depths of her subconscious to help her along in this last part of her journey. Dick and I looked at each other, and I knew from his expression the end would be soon. After Dick left, I had a talk with a few of the floor nurses, and I asked them how long it would be. It was Tuesday. Friday, they all agreed. Friday was the day. TGIF. Sure.

But then Wednesday came and Dick stopped by in the morning. "This is going to be a big day," he said to me. He couldn't say more, or else he would be sharing a cell with Jack Kevorkian, but he repeated, "This is going to be a big day." Words I never wanted to hear. So I steeled myself. April 30 was the day that would go down in infamy, the Pearl Harbor of my life, the day that my beloved wife, Karen, passed away. Her morphine level had been raised to forty. I sat beside her all day, waiting for the end. She looked so peaceful. But she kept breathing, just as she always had.

I was starving, so I took a break and went down to the awful Cedars cafeteria. I bought a creation called a Blue Bunny, an ice cream bar in the shape of a little rabbit, and I ate it, and it was good. I felt ashamed for enjoying it, while my poor Weight Watchers wife might be breathing her last at the moment. In the future, whenever I stop by the cafeteria at Cedars, I looked at those Blue Bunnies and thought of Karen. I never touched one again. I went back upstairs. Karen was still breathing. I stayed until after midnight and "the big day" was over, then went home to feed the cats and sleep another dreamless sleep, the sleep of exhaustion.

The next morning, Karen was on 60 mg of morphine. Her breathing was more restless, noisier. This had to be the day, I said to myself. I longed to speak to her, to wake her up from her drugged sleep and laugh and share some great times. But it could not be. So I sat down and wrote a farewell letter to Karen, just as she had written Doodle:

My dearest Karen,

Today is May 1. I am sitting by your bedside. You are on a morphine drip. I pray that you are in comfort. I believe that there is no more physical pain and pray that there is no mental pain or anguish at this time. I guess I should have written this before, but until the end of last week, I had hoped that the medications would work, not just to keep you alive, but to give some quality of life, whatever that means. I promised you that Dr. Helfenstein would "snow you." And he has done all that he could in these last moments. I am looking at you lying with mouth open, face tight and yellow. Everyone says how beautiful you are, and your friends know that the beauty and grace are you, your body and soul… The first time I saw you I fell in love. It was a blessing to have met you, to love you, to share joys and some sorrows together. I know that some people will say it and not mean it, but I truthfully wish it were me in that bed instead of you. You have expressed to everyone how worried you are about me when you pass on. I cannot truthfully say I will be all right, because I will not. I cannot bear the thought of being and living without you.

You are the kindest, most considerate person I have ever met. You always cared so much for the other person and really felt their pain. You tried to help as many people as you could. Needless to say, my patients loved you and I jealously shared you with them.

I went on to write about our courtship, our marriage, our wonderful life together, how she made my practice, how my patients loved her, how she believed in me from the glories of my career triumphs through the dark days of the federal witch hunt. The letter continued:

Outside of the practice, we decorated our houses together, planned our gardens, and shopped a whole lot. Our tastes in foods, clothes, furniture and style merged, as did our souls. Your mother could barely disguise her love for our children, our kittens. The Tinker, Doodle, and Wojge are in heaven now and waiting for you.

I remember how you cried in 1995 when I was diagnosed with cancer. I have a slow growing but incurable non-Hodgkins lymphoma. I told you I would be okay, but knew that 60 percent plus transform into the aggressive type and that's terminal within six to eight years. Well, this is the eighth year, and I'm still here. You were diagnosed in June 1999 and are lying in bed today, May 1, 2003, in a coma, with only a few days at most left. You had a 95 percent chance of survival until September 2000 when metastatic cancer was found. I sincerely wish it was reversed. Better yet, if death is here, better that we both die now, like Romeo and Juliet. Life is so ironic, unpredictable, and many times so unfair. Today I received your copy of Cure *magazine, and there's an article on new therapies for advanced breast cancer, with longer, better life. There's also an article on caregiving and the end of life. I can't bear to read the first article anymore. My caregiving role is just about up. And so is the end-of-life care. It does not do any good, but it hurts so much to think about how your doctors betrayed you.*

The letter continued. I went through the litany of medical atrocities that had befallen her.

I watched you in February 2003 as your liver literally exploded with cancer. The physical pain was unbearable, but you stayed through it, although, as you said then, "Do I have a choice?" Dr. Helfenstein, who at first told me you were dying, was very surprised at your fighting spirit. I was in awe of your strength and grace and cried when you apologized to the oncologist about being a difficult patient. I wish I could have washed away your fears. You told me how scared you were and knew that you were dying. My lovely Karen, how I wish I could have comforted you more. It's now 2:15 p.m., May 1, 2003. I am watching you. I love you so much. It's unbearable to watch you take your last breaths. I cannot imagine life without you. Please forgive me if I ever hurt you in any way.

And that was it.

But Karen didn't die that day. Or the next. I was disappointed that she was not out of her profound misery. Yet each morning I was overjoyed to see her breathing, to see her body still moving, to know her body was still alive, whatever that meant at this point. I was obviously conflicted. These anticlimaxes were destroying me. Dick came by. He upped Karen's morphine level to 100.

Friday morphed into Saturday. Weekends were the cruelest time to be ill, because you never know who was going to be covering for your regular doctor, who was invariably away. I was basically camped out on the cancer floor, waiting for the inevitable. Covering for Dick that weekend was a young doctor who looked more like a Malibu surfer girl than a Cedars oncologist, tall, blonde, with hair that came down as far as the shocking black leather miniskirt she was wearing. Maybe the idea was to shock the comatose patients into consciousness. Her appearance certainly shocked me. This doctor was straight out of Central Casting, a pure celluloid fantasy of a physical physician.

I had waited for about three hours that morning till the doctor had finished her rounds visiting all the patients except for Karen. She was standing at the Central Nursing Station, a very busy, impersonal, noisy and distracting area. I walked over to Dr. Surf and introduced myself as Dr. Reiter and said I'd like to talk with her in a quieter area.

"We can talk right here," she said, acting perturbed at being bothered at all.

"I'd rather sit down to discuss my wife's condition and medication schedule," I said.

Annoyed, she led the way to Karen's room. How she thought it was appropriate to discuss a dying woman's care or prognosis or treatment in front of the patient, my wife, was beyond the pale of my belief.

"Could we please sit in the quiet room?" I asked. The quiet room was a small room on the floor set aside for families to speak among themselves or their doctors, a quiet simple setting for the discussion of life-and-death issues. I wanted to remind the young doctor how to talk to patients and their families, how to break or discuss bad news. She clearly had no idea. Her body language was hostile, tense, the dramatic opposite of what I thought all doctors were supposed to know about the bedside manner protocols of death. She must have realized that as a doctor I knew the inevitable outcome. Karen was in a morphine-induced coma. I wanted to know how long this torture would go on. She had to take some time to talk to me, something she was trained to do. She had the chart and should have read it before talking to me at all. "What do you want?" was her bedside manner. What I wanted was to keep raising Karen's morphine, as Dick had been doing very discreetly.

The doctor didn't say a word. She marched into Karen's room, took her stethoscope and listened to her stomach and chest.

"I'm not raising her morphine," she said. "She seems comfortable. She's doing fine."

"Fine?" I exploded, pulling the doctor out of the room on the far off chance Karen might hear us. "She's dying of terminal cancer."

"I listened to her," Surfer Doctor said.

"Did you listen to her heart? Did you listen to her soul? How do you know if she's suffering? By that stethoscope in your ears?"

This was way too heavy for Doctor Surf. She turned and left. I was too paralyzed to fight any more. I looked back in at Karen, jaundiced, yellow, gaunt, dying. Her beauty was gone.

Sunday morning I noticed that they were still doing blood tests on Karen, who was in a deep coma, seemingly oblivious to the world she was leaving. What were these blood tests for? "It's to test her oxygen saturation in the blood," the nurse assigned to the room replied, noting Karen was on a morphine and respiratory depressant. I could not believe I was hearing this—worried about her lung function at this stage of the game? It was 62 percent, less than two-thirds of normal. Most people would be blue or cyanotic at this level, and dead, but I assumed since Karen was in a deep coma, her body could tolerate this level, but not for long.

Again, Doctor Surfer appeared, making her rounds. She popped in and asked how I was, and could she help me in any way.

"No thank you," I said politely, adding, "Her oxygen saturation is 62 percent."

Surfer Doc offered to give her oxygen.

"Oxygen?" I said. "She's not walking out of here. She is leaving in a casket. You're treating her like a specimen in a Petri dish."

Again, the Surfer Doc fled in horror, maybe back to Malibu to chill. Where, I wondered, was Jack Kevorkian when I needed him? I slumped back in a chair and stared forlornly at a blank wall as the hours rolled by.

Monday Dick returned, amazed to see Karen still alive. He upped the morphine once more. Now it was at 110 mg, and Karen remained in a coma, moaning at times. Was she that strong? Did she want to live after all? I had concluded beyond any doubt that she did not. A nice English nurse was there that day. She understood, and kept turning up the morphine throughout the day.

Tuesday the nice English nurse was gone, but Karen was still there. I couldn't believe it. That day a new woman from hospice came. She wasn't as sinister as Dr. Death, but she was a mindless, by-the-book bureaucrat. She gave me a poor-dear look, as if I were Jack Nicholson in *One Flew Over the Cuckoo's Nest.* Maybe I was out of my mind at this point, sleep deprived, starving, hating the world. I begged the hospice woman to give Karen more morphine. I begged like a desperate junkie. Naturally, she turned me down, and I turned her out, screaming at her.

On Wednesday, Karen's friend Valerie had come by to sit with her. Karen's morphine level was at 120, but I was still acting like a drug pusher, trying my hardest to score her more morphine.

Just as the nurse refused me by saying, "She doesn't need any more," Karen let out a blood-curdling moan that froze my soul.

"See! She heard you!" Valerie yelled at the nurse.

Upon hearing Karen's moan and Valerie's remarks, I lost control. I burst into tears and raced down the hall all the way to the next wing of the hospital. I found a phone and called Dick Helfenstein, and in between tears of grief and frustration, I implored him, I begged him to please take care of Karen.

"I'll take care of it," Dick assured me calmly. Karen didn't moan again, but she did keep breathing. It got to be 10 p.m. and Dick hadn't come by yet. I simply threw in the towel and went home to the cats, whose soft furry bodies and gentle purring gave me whatever modicum of comfort was left to my soul.

That morning, at one thirty in the morning, I was awakened from the deepest sleep of my life by a call from Cedars. Karen had passed away. In a daze, I dozed back off. It was a bad dream. A half hour later someone else called with the same news. And then the sitter called. And then I woke up, knowing it was true. I was too weak, too beaten, too drained, to go in. I just lay alone in bed all night, letting it sink in. At 6 a.m. I tried to get up, and got violently sick, throwing up, with chills and fever. I thought I was having a heart attack. I called a close friend and told him that Karen had just died. He immediately came over and stayed with me for six hours, during which I went into a shock-like state.

By noon I pulled myself together a bit, although I couldn't answer the phone. I had no idea what to say, what to do. But I couldn't go see Karen dead at Cedars. I called the hospital to make arrangement to transfer Karen's body to the mortuary. I was surprised at how businesslike and routine it all was. Yes, people died every day, and Cedars was used to this, but the business-as-usual aspect was too ghoulish for me to handle. I collapsed in grief.

The next day two close friends came over and took me to the mortuary. Karen looked beautiful in the casket, unreal, like movie stars are unreal when they're all fixed up, not like when you see them in the office. The yellow, jaundiced, gaunt look was gone. She was serene again, beautiful again. She looked as if she were from another era, a Raphael Madonna or maybe a Botticelli Venus. Whatever, she was no longer of this earth. She had gone to a better, kinder, more loving place. She had crossed the Rainbow Bridge to be made whole again, joining her beloved kittens, and somehow I could see her there, somewhere over the rainbow.

I remembered Karen once saying she wanted to be cremated; that she didn't like funerals and caskets and she didn't want to be a burden. She had apologized to her doctors for being a difficult patient when in fact the difficulty was the tenacious cancer. She gave the fight of a lifetime with endless optimism about the next medical or surgical breakthrough. And she did so with charm, spiritual elegance, beauty, and grace.

Two days later Karen was cremated. A few weeks later, in June, we had a memorial ceremony in our beautiful garden. June was literally busting out all over, the flowers, the birds, the California sun at its most brilliant. On one hand, I could imagine Karen speaking to me through the sweet voice of nature, singing her ode to joy, saying all's right with the world. But my world wasn't right at all. All the gorgeous music of nature couldn't bring Karen back to me. All I saw, all I felt, was a black emptiness.

A month later I got a statement from Blue Cross showing that Karen's final ten days at Cedars cost a staggering $33,000. It was money far better spent for poor people who lacked medical care. These were luxury prices for the ultimate luxury hospital, the high cost of dying in style. End-of-life care, Beverly Hills style. I had seen death at the top now, and it was no prettier than at the bottom, just a bigger waste, and, for me, a bigger tragedy. It certainly didn't make me proud of my once-scintillating medical career. The monument I was going to build to Karen, by saving her life and resurrecting my own in the process, was nothing but a tiny pile of dust in a gilded urn.

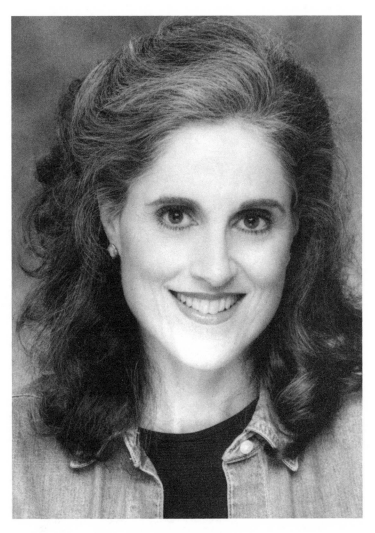

Karen – my best friend

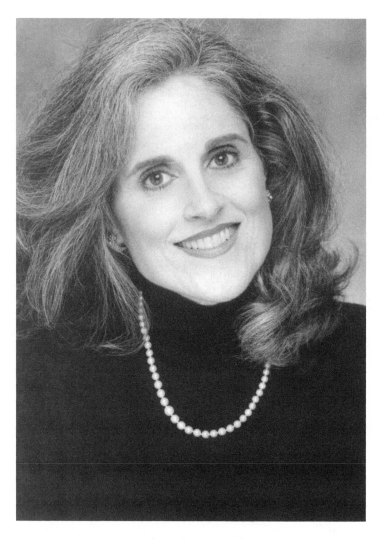

and my loving wife

EPILOGUE

For the longest time after Karen's death, I would wake up deeply surprised that I was still alive. I wasn't sure that I wanted to be.

I was bitterly angry at a medical system that had hideously betrayed both Karen and me, a system that probably sped her to an unnecessary death and certainly did nothing to ease her dying. But it was also a system in which I was a charter member.

My anger at the arrogance and ineptitudes of many of the doctors who treated Karen has not abated, and I still compose angry letters to them in my head. To share the same profession with physicians who do not care about their patients makes the doctor in me simply feel ashamed.

Eli Wiesel wisely stated, "Whoever survives a test, whatever it may be, must tell the story. That is his duty." This is our story. To tell the story is my way of healing, to tell the story of a life that has passed, of what happened to Karen, to help others in their crises of loss and to relate the moments of light and hope. In the telling of my story, I share what is most precious to me.

Twelve days after Karen died, I had a call from Sylvan Minsky, the UCLA breast cancer pathologist. Ironically, Dr. Minsky, for all his troubles at UCLA with the short-sighted research committee and the veterinarian department, left to chair the department of pathology at a large Midwestern university and prestigious medical school, where his efforts to create a vaccine for metastatic breast cancer continue. His work holds tremendous promise. Karen's metastatic liver cancer and Dr.

Minsky may one day win a Nobel Prize for a lifesaving vaccine. One day, patients all over the world may thank Karen for saving their lives.

As for me, I ask myself where am I heading with my career and without Karen.

The work that I did in my career was very challenging and that was my elixir of life—to be challenged intellectually and creatively as a surgeon. It was a passion and I felt there was no other way. I was always committed to doing the best for my patients and the best for my wife. I have begun to return to my work by observing and assisting in surgeries. Every surgery I observe, or that I assist in, brings the thrill of that career back to me. It sounds corny, but it makes me born again.

In time, I look forward to fulfilling a commitment to work here at home in free clinics and abroad with programs like The Smile Team for cleft, lip, and palate deformities, and with Doctors Without Borders, helping those around the world who have suboptimal, if any, care.

At the same time that I turn my sights toward some degree of restoration of my plastic surgery career, I continue to focus on life's lessons learned.

I feel Karen is still here, close, watching, proud of me, as she always was. Nowhere was she closer than in our garden, the garden that was so dear to her. Every time I stepped outside into that glorious garden, I see her. A vision in a straw hat with ribbons and flowers, and, as a counterpoint to that elegant, delicate hat, no-nonsense garden shoes and an apron holding shears and pruners. I see her orange tabby helper cat Tinker scampering alongside her. That was Karen, beautiful and practical, delicate and charming, a source of loveliness, a source of life. And now I am filled with sadness that she died like one of the ephemeral annual flowers.

I remember our first garden: we transformed a barren landscape into a multi-terraced English cottage garden that noted gardeners such as Gertrude Jekyll or Vita Sackville-West would have been proud of creating.

I thus got the inspiration to plant and create a new garden to remember Karen by. I found a place several levels down in our multi-layered space that we called the shade garden, with trees that let in filtered light and ivy covering the ground. In this sanctuary I wanted to experience the deepest sense of peace, peace with my past, acceptance of the loss of Karen and the loneliness I felt. And maybe forgiveness of those who hurt us, including some who did so without ever knowing.

I chose to create a Zen garden. Zen is a Japanese word that is derived from the Chinese word Ch'an, meaning meditation. Zen is a path to enlightenment, to understanding; I wanted to impart a sense of order and a spirit of tranquility and calm. I wasn't trying to excite the senses with an explosive profusion of color and sweet smelling odors; our big garden took care of that.

It was with love and care that I designed this garden, as Zen Buddhism requires that every task be performed with love. The garden put me in touch with the elements. First, I chose to include water. Without water there can be no life. I created a cool reflecting pool that reflected the surrounding shrubbery that I planted and imparted balance and ease.

This small pond was lined by another element, small stones and rocks. Rocks, with their untouched natural shape, bestow strength and character. While the world evolves in tempestuous ways, rocks remain resolute and strong. Placing these stones in certain ways harmonized them with the surrounding area.

The plants were different colors, shapes, and sizes, but the dominant color was green—the entire range of green shades and tones were used with a profusion of ferns, ivy, mosses, and exotic leafed plants such as hostas, zebras, prayer plants, African Mask, elephant ears, and succulents. I added dashes of color using baby fuchsia, bromeliads, and ti plants.

Overhead there is a canopy of ficus, pitosporum, acacia, bamboo, and jacaranda trees, which allow the sunlight to gently illuminate the ground below. For the entrance to the Zen garden, I purchased a very old bronze statue of a water girl, a life-size beauty carrying two buckets of water on a yoke. It was timeless and had an antique green patina. The water girl bears an uncanny likeness to Karen and shares her grace. Stone pathways lead to this place of contemplation and quietness. Each leaf, each blade of grass, is a type of sanctuary, a place of refuge and protection, a sacred plea that comforts me and deepens my connection to Karen as it deepens my connection to life.

It may be true that coming through a great sorrow can make us stronger and teach us what is really important. But to survive the death of a loved one is no guarantee of greater wisdom. I also became embittered and reclusive. That's when I needed friends, communities of faith, and professional help. If I can weather the storm, I hope to have a better sense of who I am and what I want most in life. I have learned to savor and cherish cool water, sunshine and wind, the smell of roses, the purring of cats, and the love and friendship I have now.

To plant a garden is to believe in tomorrow.

I continue to plant.